A clinical guide to sleep disorders in children
and adolescents

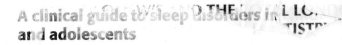

Sleep disturbance is commonplace and causes much personal distress to sufferers and their
families. It is implicated in a variety of problems, from poor educational performance or
disturbed behaviour to accidents or physical dysfunction. Traditionally, research into sleep
disorders has generally been undertaken within separate, unconnected medical disciplines and
has mainly involved adults. As sleep disturbance is closely associated with serious problems,
identifying and treating sleep disorders early is essential for good long-term health and
well-being. Yet there is no up-to-date, comprehensive, one-stop source of information for
clinicians concerning sleep disorders in young people. Gregory Stores addresses this need with
a cross-disciplinary account of available clinical information and treatments, illustrated by
actual cases of sleep problems in the young. This book will be essential reading for all
professionals involved in child healthcare from infancy to adolescence, and will also be
invaluable to general readers looking for up-to-the-minute information and references.

Gregory Stores is Professor of Developmental Neuropsychiatry in the University of Oxford.
He is an internationally recognized authority in the field of sleep disturbance in the young,
and has developed clinical services and methods of investigation in clinical neurophysiology
for children that are now in use all over the world.

A clinical guide to sleep disorders in children and adolescents

Gregory Stores

Professor of Developmental Neuropsychiatry, University of Oxford

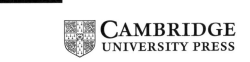

CAMBRIDGE
UNIVERSITY PRESS

PUBLISHED BY THE PRESS SYNDICATE OF THE UNIVERSITY OF CAMBRIDGE
The Pitt Building, Trumpington Street, Cambridge, United Kingdom

CAMBRIDGE UNIVERSITY PRESS
The Edinburgh Building, Cambridge CB2 2RU, UK
40 West 20th Street, New York, NY 10011-4211, USA
10 Stamford Road, Oakleigh, VIC 3166, Australia
Ruiz do Alarcón 13, 28014 Madrid, Spain
Dock House, The Waterfront, Cape Town 8001, South Africa

http://www.cambridge.org

First published 2001

Printed in the United Kingdom at the University Press, Cambridge

Typeface Minion 10.5/14pt   *System* Poltype® [v n]

A catalogue record for this book is available from the British Library

Library of Congress Cataloguing in Publication data

Stores, Gregory.
A Clinical Guide to Sleep Disorders in Children and Adolescents / Gregory Stores.
   p.   cm.
Includes bibliographical references and index.
ISBN 0 521 65398 3 (paperback)
1. Sleep disorders in children.   2. Health behaviour in adolescence.   3. Sleep.   I Title.
[DNLM: 1. Sleep Disorders – Adolescence.   2. Sleep Disorders – Child.   3. Sleep
Disorders – Infant. WM 188 S884c 2001]
RJ506.5.S55 S865 2001
618.92'8498–dc21   00-060803

ISBN 0 521 65398 3 paperback

Every effort has been made in preparing this book to provide accurate and up-to-date information which is in accord with accepted standards and practice at the time of publication. Nevertheless, the author, editors and publisher can make no warranties that the information contained herein is totally free from error, not least because clinical standards are constantly changing through research and regulation. The author, editors and publisher therefore disclaim all liability for direct or consequential damages resulting from the use of material contained in this book. Readers are strongly advised to pay careful attention to information provided by the manufacturer of any drugs or equipment that they plan to use.

   Although case histories are drawn from actual cases, every effort has been made to disguise the identities of the individuals involved.

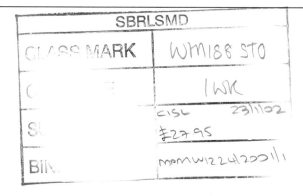

Contents

Acknowledgements

I have been fortunate in recent years to have had the opportunity to realize a longstanding ambition to concentrate on clinical and academic aspects of the fascinating field of sleep disorders and, with the help of colleagues, to bring it to the attention of child healthcare professionals. The appeal of 'sleep disorders medicine' lies to a large extent on its relevance to many people, its importance for child development in particular, and its cross-specialty and interdisciplinary nature.

A number of people have helped to formulate my own approach to the sleep disorders field, but I am especially indebted to Luci Wiggs who has been a vital and much appreciated influence, both clinically and in our various joint research endeavours.

I am also grateful to those who, in addition to Luci, commented on the drafts of this book, namely Harvey Markovitch, Rebecca Stores and Anne Thomson.

Finally, I wish to thank my wife, Christina, for helping to produce the various drafts of the book with speed, accuracy, constructive comment and much forbearance.

Children's sleep disorders: a case of serious neglect

There can be few more striking examples of the gap between clinical need and provision of services than sleep disorders medicine, especially concerning children. Sleep problems are endemic and yet their recognition, diagnosis and treatment constitute a blind spot in medical and other healthcare education. The scope and importance of sleep disorders medicine is grossly underestimated by the limited (often perfunctory) accounts of children's sleep and its disorders in textbooks of paediatrics and child psychiatry.

In clinical practice, major errors are made in all the main categories of sleep disturbance. Sleeplessness is frequently treated symptomatically without considering the underlying cause; excessive sleepiness is commonly misconstrued as laziness or some other form of psychological shortcoming; and the many types of episodic disturbances of behaviour associated with sleep are regularly confused with each other diagnostically. The consequences to patients and their families of these mistakes are inevitably serious.

There are several reasons for this unfortunate state of affairs. One major factor must be the wide-ranging nature of the study of sleep and its disorders which crosses many of the boundaries between conventional disciplines and medical specialties. This poses problems for the more traditional teaching and training programmes where learning and the acquisition of skills are still confined to separate compartments with little attempt at integration. In this setting, multidisciplinary areas of discourse and clinical practice are likely to be poorly represented. This is especially so with the ever-increasing pressure on professional curricula, particularly in medicine in view of the spectacular advances in molecular medicine, imaging techniques and other technologically sophisticated and prestigious fields.

Sleep disorders medicine is likely to make increasing use of such impressive advances but, as a specialty, it has difficulty competing for time in teaching courses, especially in view of its unfamiliarity to teaching programme planners. The scientific study of sleep and its disorders is very recent and with the emphasis still firmly on adults. Indeed, reviews of the history of sleep disorders medicine hardly mention children at all. It is a tribute to the imagination and diligence of both basic and clinical sleep researchers that so much information has accumulated in such a short period of time. However, the imbalance remains, with children's sleep disorders medicine still under-represented in clinical practice and research.

A more fundamental reason why sleep problems are not taken sufficiently seriously by professionals may be the supposed basic familiarity of such problems. Everyone experiences difficulties with their sleep at some time or other. Usually, the problem is short-lived and more a nuisance than anything more serious. Many parents are only too familiar with their young child's refusal to go to bed at the required time, or being woken in the night for attention. This is easily seen as part of the mixed blessing of parenthood and something to be endured until matters (hopefully) improve. In other words, there may be a common feeling that sleep problems do not merit a great deal of professional attention compared with other difficulties. This rather casual approach to sleep problems appears to be quite widespread.

In fact, any such attitude flies in the face of the evidence that, at all ages, sleep disturbance is the cause of much suffering, disadvantage and risk. This claim does not rest simply on the overvalued idea of sleep disorders medicine enthusiasts, it is supported, for example, by the closely argued case for more educational and clinical interest and more research funding presented to the US Government in the Wake Up America documents (National Commission on Sleep Disorders Research 1993, 1994).

A main point in these and less extensive accounts to the same effect (such as Dement & Mitler, 1993), is that persistent sleep disturbance often causes much personal distress, poor educational and occupational performance, and social and recreational difficulties. It is also implicated in many types of accident, including man-made disasters. Physical- and mental-health problems may also result. The cost to the national economy is considered to be huge. There is no reason to believe that the impact of sleep disorders is any less than universal, or that adverse effects are confined to adults on whom, again, emphasis has been placed in these publications.

These facts need to be brought home to the public and professionals alike. Those suffering from sleep disturbance (and their relatives) should be encouraged to recognize that such problems are not only troublesome but potentially serious, and that effective treatment (if based on accurate diagnosis of the underlying cause) can be available. The idea that medication is the only available treatment needs to be corrected and the value of psychological treatments more widely known. Raised public expectations that help should and can be available would act as a spur to the better provision of clinical services for sleep problems. This, in turn, would require better training for providers of those services. The basic need is better education all round.

Despite the quite entrenched reasons why sleep disorders medicine has been a Cinderella specialty, optimism that matters will improve is justified. It is the experience of teachers in the field that the topic is invariably interesting to audiences, whether lay or professional. Those with a sleep problem of their own, parents and other relatives, teachers, medical students, neurologists, paediatricians, psychiatrists and psychologists invariably want to know more when sleep and its disorders is presented as the intriguing subject that it is, with important practical and clinical aspects, as well as many research possibilities.

This demand for further information is only partially met at the present time. The neglect of sleep and its disorders in professional education has been a self-perpetuating problem with relatively few enthusiasts (capable of enthusing others) entering the field. However, a trend towards more professionals from various backgrounds developing a special interest in the area is evident from the increasing membership of national and international sleep societies and the establishment of new national groups.

A number of textbooks, published in recent years, will have made their own contribution to increased awareness of and knowledge about the sleep disorders field, although their main appeal seems likely to have been to those already specially interested in the subject. Books written for sufferers themselves and relatives have also been a welcome development. The present text is intended to fill the gap between books for professionals with a specialized interest in children's sleep disorders and those written for parents. It emphasizes practical approaches to the recognition, diagnosis and treatment of sleep disorders in infancy, childhood and adolescence, and is intended to be useful mainly to paediatricians, psychiatrists, psychologists and others who are professionally concerned with child health and welfare.

To maintain the essentially clinical rather than academic nature of the text, referencing is restricted. However, sources of more detailed information are cited in the form of selected review articles and chapters, together with more specific publications to supplement or update the more general accounts, or to emphasize certain points. Heavily technical accounts of limited appeal to the nonspecialist reader have been avoided. Personal clinical impressions are also included on aspects which have not been the subject of empirical research.

For the most part, the references chosen are concerned with studies or observations on children or adolescents, but some reports on adults are included where the content seems likely also to be relevant to younger patients. The case histories throughout the book are drawn from the author's own clinical practice, preserving the anonymity of each child and family. Although the patients have mainly attended a special sleep disorders clinic, the basic principles that they illustrate, and the treatment approaches described, are relevant to children with sleep disorders in general, seen typically in non-specialized clinical services. *The main aim is to provide the reader who does not have a specialized interest in sleep disorders with an overview and a suggested clinical approach to the many conditions covered in children's sleep disorders medicine.* The fine details of treatments are not attempted but can be found in the references cited. Necessarily, many statements are subject to revision in the light of further research.

In places, the child is referred to as 'he' purely for convenience. The layout adopted, with bullet points and other subdivisions, is intended to facilitate access to the information contained in the text.

Chapter 2 consists of a more detailed account of the main general points made in these opening comments.

General issues

History of sleep disorders in children and adolescents

Those of an historical inclination might be interested in the provenance of present-day practice and research in children's sleep disorders. There is, in fact, not much to say, and what can be said is a patchwork of historical, literary and clinical references which illustrates that children's sleep disorders have long been recognized but without any systematic study until recent times.

The starting-point might best be described as 'prescientifically paediatric'. In *The Boke of Chyldren* (1545), Thomas Phaire included in his list of 'the manye grevous and perilous diseases' with which children of his day were afflicted 'terrible dreames and feare in the slepe' (caused by 'the arysing of stynkyng vapours out of yᵉ stomake into the fantasye, and sences of the brayne') and also 'pissing in the bedde'. To what extent Phaire's suggested remedies would meet the requirements of present-day evidence-based practice is doubtful. For example, his observations of childhood nightmares were accurate, but the treatments he recommended included 'a lytle pouder of the seedes of peonie and sometimes triacle'. 'The poudered wesande [windpipe] of a cocke' and 'the stones of an hedgehogge poudred' were some of his recommendations for bedwetting.

To do justice to Phaire, it must be said that at least he was drawing attention to the special medical problems of the young at a time when, in general, few if any concessions were made to children, who were viewed as small adults and dealt with accordingly (Pinchbeck & Hewitt, 1969). Just as childhood is a relatively new concept, paediatrics has largely been emancipated from general medicine only recently. Examples remain, in the provision of various clinical services, of inadequate acknowledgment of the special needs of children.

Some of the best early clinical descriptions of sleep disorders are available in the novels of Charles Dickens. Cosnett (1992) has discussed how Dickens took an interest in sleep problems, possibly because of his own insomnia. He described them in several of his characters in such detail that they must have been based on real people. The best-known example is the Fat Boy Joe in *Pickwick Papers* (Dickens, 1836/7). The usual diagnosis of Joe's excessive sleepiness is obstructive sleep apnoea, although his obesity (seen in only the minority of children with this condition), overeating and periodic behavioural disturbance raises other possibilities, notably the Kleine–Levin syndrome.

The short history of the scientific study of sleep and sleep disorders has been described by Thorpy (2000). Significantly, this and other historical accounts contain little about children and adolescents. It is the case, however, that some time ago the Stanford University group drew attention to the clinical importance of sleepiness in children and chided physicians for usually not taking any interest in the problem until significant complications had arisen (Anders et al., 1978). In fact, there had been a much earlier warning about the potentially serious effects on young schoolchildren of lack of sleep. The anxieties expressed by Dukes (1905) were overdramatic, but his concerns anticipated similar warnings expressed by later writers. He complained that 'younger pupils are all offered the same number of hours as the seniors for sleep. What this means to children is lowered vitality, apathy, bloodlessness, and diminished growth of body and brain. It renders the child an easy prey to disease, and causes slight fainting attacks resembling those cases of epilepsy termed petit mal.' Not a great deal of notice has been taken of Dukes nor, indeed, Anders and his colleagues, except, to some extent, regarding the common problem of sleepiness in adolescence which became the special interest of Dement and Carskadon at Stanford (Dement, 1990).

As mentioned already, there has been a determined attempt more recently (especially in the USA) to bring to public, professional and governmental attention the importance of sleep disorders in adults, but with little mention of children in whom sleep problems are common and for whose development persistent sleep disruption can be expected to have particularly important implications. The International Classification of Sleep Disorders (American Sleep Disorders Association, 1997) is essentially adult based. It contains limited recognition of the differences between adults and children (discussed later) in the pattern of occurrence of sleep disorders, the way basically the same condition can present itself clinically or physiologically, and the different implications for psychological and sometimes physical development.

That is not to say that much is not already known of considerable clinical importance and research interest regarding children (Ferber & Kryger, 1995). There is still an urgent need to incorporate this knowledge widely into clinical practice and to pursue answers to the questions and uncertainties that remain concerning the nature and consequences for young people of the many ways in which sleep can be disturbed.

Prevalence of children's sleep disorders in the general population

Because of failures of recognition and limited referral of cases for medical attention, it is not known with accuracy how many people of any age suffer from sleep disorders. Much greater awareness and diagnostic sophistication are required before reliable figures can be expected. In the meantime, it is reasonable to assume that the usually quoted figures are underestimations. Even so, there is ample evidence that sleep disorders are very common.

Overall, it seems likely that at least 20–30% of children from infancy to adolescence have sleep problems that are considered significant by them or their parents (Mindell, 1993). Intriguingly, the pattern of reported problems can vary from one nation to another according to a survey of 11–16-year-olds in eleven European countries (Tynjälä et al., 1993).

Perhaps the most reliable figures for more specific sleep problems are those based on population studies of settling and night-waking problems in toddlers, about 20–25% of whom pose such problems to their parents most nights and sometimes every night (Richman, 1987). The importance of collecting information from more than one source about the occurrence of sleep problems is illustrated in the survey of sleep habits and sleep disturbance in 4–11-year-old children by Owens et al. (2000). By using a battery of sleep questionnaires for parents, teachers and children themselves, it was possible to identify a range of types of sleep disturbance some of which might well have been missed if only parental information had been collected.

Severe sleep problems show a further high occurrence rate in adolescence, including those due to erratic sleep–wake patterns and the delayed sleep phase syndrome (DSPS) (see later) which causes a combination of inability to get off to sleep and great difficulty getting up in the morning. Although at a lower level, the reported prevalence rates for some other conditions causing excessive daytime sleepiness in young people also illustrate that these disorders are by no means the rarities that might be supposed. For example, upper airway obstruction during sleep is said to occur in about 2% of children from infancy onwards (Carroll & Loughlin, 1995a). If the suggested prevalence estimates for narcolepsy (4–6 per 10,000 in the United States) are correct, then the rate of this disorder in children and adolescents must be at least a third of this figure because of the general agreement that the first symptoms frequently appear at this early age (Stores, 1999a).

Prevalence rates for the third main type of childhood sleep problem (i.e. in addition to sleeplessness and excessive sleepiness), namely episodes of disturbed behaviour associated with sleep (the parasomnias), are difficult to judge. Only a small proportion seem to come to medical attention, partly because some occur infrequently in perhaps the majority of children. Accurate prevalence rates are also made difficult to obtain by the fact that different parasomnias are often not distinguished from each other very clearly, with a tendency to use the term 'nightmare' for any that involves dramatic changes of behaviour. Again, it seems that the frequency with which children are seen professionally for help with this type of sleep disturbance is no guide to the occurrence of such problems in the community at large.

Children at high risk of sleep disturbance (Stores & Wiggs, 2001)

Sleep disturbance is common enough in children in general, but some groups are particularly prone, namely certain children with various types of physical or psychological disorder including those with a learning disability (mental retardation). However, there are some subgroups within the general population who are at special risk because of developmental factors.

General population

Some of the changes in sleep physiology in the period between infancy and adult life may predispose children to sleep disorders at certain stages of development. Other important changes having the same effect concern parenting or changes in life style.

- Rapid Eye Movement (REM) sleep is prominent in *early infancy*, possibly explaining in part why sleep seems to be fragile then as this type of sleep is less sound than nonREM (NREM) sleep.
- In the *toddler years* a basic aspect of parenting is to establish satisfactory sleep patterns. Failure to do so is common, resulting mainly in settling and night-waking problems in 20% or more of children of this age.
- Deep NREM sleep is particularly prominent in *early childhood*. This may be a reason why arousal disorders (such as sleepwalking), which arise from this form of sleep, occur mainly at this age.
- In contrast, the amount of slow wave sleep (SWS) decreases in *adolescence*. Of apparently greater importance, however, is that (out of keeping with the progressive decline at earlier ages) sleep requirements do not decrease at puberty. Also, the overnight sleep phase becomes delayed partly for biological reasons, judging by the fact that the extent of the delay is related to stage of puberty and that the timing of melatonin secretion changes in early adolescence in relation to this sleep-phase delay (Carskadon et al., 1997). Increasingly, as adolescence progresses, these physiological factors, combined with strong social influences (e.g. to stay up late especially at weekends) frequently cause sleep deprivation, daytime sleepiness and various adverse effects on mood, behaviour and performance (Carskadon, 1990).

The complex origins of the particularly high rates of sleep disturbance seen in adolescence illustrate the need to discover more about the psychosocial and other factors which put certain groups of children at particular risk of serious sleep disturbance and its consequences.

In general, current information about the origins of children's sleep difficulties is only preliminary. Infant's sleep problems are the most researched (Sadeh & Anders, 1993). A number of important biological factors including perinatal complications and temperament have been implicated, as well as socioeconomic factors such as overcrowding. Parenting practices and standards are obviously relevant, and also parental psychiatric illness (Seifer et al., 1996). However, outside grossly distorted or abnormal circumstances, precise prediction of which infants will develop serious sleep problems is difficult because of the many interacting influences involved. As will be mentioned later, relatively subtle factors have been suggested by recent research, such as mothers' attitudes and emotional reactions to their children's sleep patterns, perhaps based partly on their own experience of sleep as infants or their feelings of competence as parents (Morrell, 1999). Insight into such influences might explain why objectively the same degree of sleep disturbance is seen as a serious problem by some parents and not at all by others.

Chronic physical illness, disorder or disability

As part of being generally unwell, or because of discomfort or distress, acute illness usually affects sleep, mainly for the duration of the illness although the experience of being ill, receiving treatment or being *admitted to hospital* (White et al., 1990) can cause a sleep disturbance which persists for some time afterwards. For example, this has been described in children who have undergone intensive care, even for a relatively short period (Cureton-Lane & Fontaine, 1997).

It is difficult to think of any chronic disorder which is not complicated by long-standing sleep disturbance. It seems, however, that this is often overlooked because the physical aspects of the condition occupy the attention of those caring for the child. Parents may share this preoccupation, or consider that the sleep problem is inevitable and untreatable which is rarely true. Failure to identify and treat a child's sleep problems may well mean that the opportunity is missed to improve his overall well-being (and that of his carers) and to help him to cope with the other difficulties imposed by the basic condition.

Sleep may be disturbed by physical conditions in various ways.

- Examples of the effects of *night-time discomfort or pain* include severe atopic dermatitis (Stores et al., 1998d), juvenile rheumatoid arthritis (Zamir et al., 1998) and malignancy (Miser et al., 1987). Pain is, in fact, related to sleep disturbance and its possible psychological and physical consequences in a number of ways (Lewin & Dahl, 1999). These include direct adverse effects on the duration and quality of sleep and the influence on sleep of the emotional upset caused by the painful condition. This is well illustrated in the consequences of burn injury where sleep disturbance can be very persistent (Lawrence et al., 1998). Promotion of better sleep is likely to improve the child's ability to cope with illness and possibly to hasten recovery from it (Adam & Oswald, 1984).

• *Some disorders worsen at night.* For example, this happens in asthma (possibly more often than usually supposed) in which the main sleep disruption appears to be frequent awakenings for variable lengths of time including brief periods which are likely to be undetected clinically (Stores et al., 1998c). The worsening of respiratory function in asthma (and also in bronchopulmonary dysplasia and cystic fibrosis) has been discussed by Loughlin and Carroll (1995). Childhood epilepsies, even in relatively mild form, are associated with high rates of sleep complaints, especially those suggesting poor quality of overnight sleep (Stores et al., 1998e). In some cases the cause appears to be nocturnal seizures, but other factors are also likely to be responsible, such as the underlying cause of the epilepsy and the accompanying psychological problems of many children with epilepsy (Cortesi et al., 1999).

• As will be discussed later, sleep disturbance caused by *upper-airway obstruction* (*UAO*) at night is reported to be common in the general population but it is particularly associated with a range of specific disorders. Main examples of this is learning disability (discussed shortly) and also some forms of cerebral palsy (Kotagal et al., 1994), neuromuscular disorders (Attarian, 2000), craniofacial abnormalities (Hoeve et al., 1999), myelomeningocele (Kirk et al., 1999), achondroplasia (Tasker et al., 1998) and sickle cell disease (Samuels et al., 1992). UAO has been implicated in the final events leading to sudden infant death syndrome (cot death) although the factors, including sleep mechanisms, leading to this dramatic outcome have yet to be made clear (Cornwell, 1995).

• *Sensory impairment* can affect sleep in different ways. Severe visual impairment is likely to lead to circadian sleep–wake cycle disorders because light perception is the main cue to establishing and maintaining a normal 24-hour sleep–wake pattern. However, other types of sleep disturbance, both physical and behavioural in origin, can also be expected in visually impaired children in view of the diversity regarding the cause of their condition and also comorbidity (Stores & Ramchandani, 1999). The very limited research on children with a hearing impairment suggests they also have a range of sleep disorders apparently including circadian sleep–wake cycle abnormalities (Oishibashie et al., 1993). Accompanying conditions, such as tinnitus (Rizzardo et al., 1998) or psychological disturbance (Roberts & Hindley, 1999), are likely to affect sleep.

CASE: A 2-year-old girl with septo-optic dysplasia and diabetes insipidus was referred by her family doctor who said that 'her appreciation of day and night was totally disrupted' causing her mother to be 'at her wit's end'. She was said to have been a restless sleeper as an infant but by 9 months of age her sleep at night was interrupted by drinking and wetting repeatedly because of diabetes insipidus. This responded quite well to treatment with dDAVP. At the time of referral her sleep was said to be very variable in duration and timing including day–night reversal. Hypnotic medication had not helped.

Magnetic resonance imaging (MRI) showed an absent septum pellucidum, with small optic nerves, chiasm and optic tracts. In addition there was evidence of cerebral cortical dysplasia in the region of the right Sylvian fissure and left temporal lobe, and the hypothalamus was reported as being abnormally small. Developmental assessment suggested that the child was of normal overall ability. She attended a mainstream nursery but was said to be sometimes too tired to join in activities there.

The results of a sleep diary, completed over a 4-week period, demonstrated a highly disorganized and variable sleep–wake schedule, with frequent daytime naps at irregular times and night-time sleep similarly broken into several short periods.

Initial attempts to produce a more regular sleep–wake pattern consisted of encouraging a regular routine for sleeping, meals and all other activities and making maximum use of nonvisual cues for entraining the circadian sleep–wake pattern. This significantly consolidated her sleep at night (although with some interruptions caused by persistent nocturia) and her daytime sleep periods became fewer. The new routine involves mother rocking the child to sleep and allowing her to sleep in her bed. It is hoped that this dependence on mother's company at night can be gradually eliminated.

Depending on progress, light therapy will be tried on the basis that some blind people seem to be still sensitive to light cues for setting their sleep–wake cycle, possibly because a collateral visual pathway from the retina to the suprachiasmatic nuclei may remain intact even when there is no sight (Czeisler et al., 1995). Melatonin could be another form of treatment (see chapter 3) but the details of its use would need to be carefully considered.

Comment: This case illustrates that both physical and behavioural factors may well need to be considered in explaining the sleep problems of children with a neurological disorder. Parenting influences are often important in such cases, including high levels of concern, but it should be possible to change them to improve the child's sleep pattern by means of a comprehensive approach.

- The *breakdown of immune systems* in human immunodeficiency virus (HIV) infected children is associated with prominent sleep–wake disturbances comparable to those described in affected adults (Franck et al., 1999).
- In *other forms of chronic illness* (endocrine, renal or hepatic, for example) the various ways in which sleep is disturbed appear to be part of the general systemic disturbance. The precise mechanisms involved are unclear, as in the disrupted sleep physiology reported in children with diabetes mellitus (Matyka et al., 2000).
- Some types of paediatric *medication* have a reputation for disturbing sleep

although, again, the details are unclear and individual differences seem to be prominent. Theophylline has this reputation which, however, has not been particularly confirmed by research on children taking this medication for asthma (Avital et al., 1991). Its potentially direct sleep-disrupting effects may, in any case, be more than outweighed by its beneficial respiratory action resulting in improved sleep.

Disturbed sleep was considered a risk with the older antiepileptic drugs especially the barbiturates which, like the benzodiazepines used in seizure control, can also cause daytime sleepiness. Abnormal drowsiness has been associated with the chronic use of some other antiepileptic drugs (Salinsky, 1996) but it can be difficult to disentangle possible direct effects of medication and underlying cerebral pathology. The possibility of a coexisting sleep disorder should also be considered (Malow et al., 1997). In fact, sleep can generally be expected to improve when seizures are controlled (Rosen et al., 1982). The sleep effects of the newer antiepileptic drugs are not well documented and should be considered. For example, a severe form of insomnia has been described in some adult patients taking lamotrigine (Sadler, 1999).

Other treatments (usually prescribed but sometimes bought over the counter) with reported adverse effects on sleep and wakefulness include antihistamines, antiemetics, anorectics, corticosteroids, cytotoxic drugs and analgesics (Nicholson et al., 1994; Obermeyer & Benca, 1996). The relative contribution of drug treatment to the sleep problems of acquired immune deficiency syndrome (AIDS) sufferers has also been considered (Phillips, 1999).

Learning disability (mental retardation)

Very high rates have been consistently described in children with a learning disability whose problems are often severe, long-standing and poorly managed (Stores, 1992). Of course, the term 'learning disability' (the currently preferred term in the UK for what elsewhere would be called mental retardation or perhaps intellectual disability) covers a very wide range of conditions which differ greatly in terms of their aetiology, severity and associated problems. Not surprisingly, therefore, most general statements about the sleep problems of learning disabled children are not valid. Some sleep problems are clearly behavioural in the sense of being mainly the result of permissive, inconsistent or otherwise unhelpful parenting practices; others are the result of physical aspects of the child's basic condition. As illustrated by the last case, there may well be a combination of reasons why the child sleeps badly.

There has been interest in the possibility that some forms of sleep disturbance are specifically part of the 'behavioural phenotype' of certain learning disability conditions such as the Smith–Magenis syndrome in which prominent sleep disturbance is described, sometimes taking the form of particularly distressed waking during the night (Colley et al., 1990). Sleeping difficulties are usually also cited as part of the characteristic clinical picture of Williams syndrome (Udwin et al., 1987) in which disruption of sleep by periodic limb movements has been reported (Arens et al., 1998). The possibility that focal brain lesions might contribute significantly to the sleep disturbances of patients with Norrie disease, Prader–Willi syndrome and Moebius syndrome has been discussed by Parkes (1999). However, assessment of the specificity of such features (and other reported phenotypical characteristics) will require much further research of a sophisticated type (Flint, 1996).

Upper airway obstruction during sleep, as well as other sleep disorders, features prominently in various learning disability conditions such as Down syndrome (Silverman, 1988) in which parental reports of their children's sleep problems show a distinctive pattern suggestive of sleep-related breathing problems compared to children with other forms of learning disability (Stores et al., 1996). Similar breathing problems at night are reported in the mucopolysaccharidoses (Bax & Colville, 1995) and the fragile-X syndrome (Tirosh & Borochowitz, 1992) although other sleep disorders have been described in children with this condition (Hagerman et al., 1995). Sometimes they also account for the excessive sleepiness seen in the Prader–Willi syndrome, although the origins of the sleep disturbance in this condition are complex (Richdale et al., 1999). Severe sleep problems are also widely reported in children with other chronic neurological disorders such as Rett syndrome (McArthur & Budden, 1998) and Angelman syndrome (Clayton-Smith, 1993).

CASE: An 8-year-old boy was referred by his paediatrician for advice about his increasingly disturbed behaviour at night. He had shown signs of severe global developmental delay from an early age. The combination of this, a generally happy and affectionate disposition during the day despite being somewhat overactive, facial features suggestive of the syndrome and characteristic EEG findings led to a diagnosis of Angelman syndrome.

In contrast to daytime, his behaviour at night was extremely disruptive. He was said to have had difficulty settling to sleep since infancy, but in recent years he was very reluctant to settle, jumping up and down and screaming for at least an hour after being put to bed. When eventually settled, he would sleep for only about 4 hours before becoming very disturbed again for about 2 hours and then sleeping for only another few hours. Repeated attempts to improve his sleep with medication had been unsuccessful. Behavioural treatment had not been feasible because of the family's overall difficulties in coping with the situation and implementing a treatment programme.

In view of the recent report of its effectiveness in children with Angelman syndrome (Zhdanova et al., 1999), a low dose of melatonin at bedtime was recommended which was soon followed by a distinct improvement in the night waking and general level of night-time disturbance.

Comment: Improvement seemed convincingly a response to melatonin treatment in this case because no other change in the circumstances was evident at the time it was used. However, as discussed in chapter 3, the overall place of melatonin in the treatment of sleep disorders is difficult to judge at the present time, mainly for lack of adequately designed research on its use.

Comorbid conditions contributing to disturbed sleep are likely to be present in many of these disorders. Epilepsy is a common accompaniment. It is closely linked, for example, to the sleep problems of children with tuberous sclerosis (Hunt & Stores, 1994). Physical disability can cause discomfort in bed (Burton, 1990). Sensory impairments or behavioural disturbance, which are common complications, also predispose affected children to sleep disturbance.

Contrary to the belief of some professionals and parents, at least the behavioural types of sleep disorder in learning-disabled children can be treated very effectively (Lancioni et al., 1999). The idea that sleep disturbance is an inevitable and untreatable part of having a disabled child should be discouraged, because good results are as possible with such children as with others who are not disabled. Perhaps especially for disabled children, it is essential that treatment programmes are individually designed in the light of the particular needs and capabilities of the family, and that they are pursued consistently and with conviction. Otherwise, parents become discouraged and conclude that their suspicions that there is no effective treatment are confirmed.

Treatment of the physical causes of sleep disturbance in this group of children may be difficult for anatomical reasons, but various possibilities (admittedly in need of further evaluation) do exist. Examples are the use of mechanical measures or surgical correction of upper-airway obstruction caused by congenital abnormalities of the upper airway structures (Carroll & Loughlin, 1995b).

CASE: A 3-year-old girl had suffered severe perinatal birth asphyxia causing spastic quadriparesis, epilepsy and global developmental delay. She was said to have always cried a lot especially at night when she was put down to sleep. In the last nine months this problem had worsened and, in addition, she woke repeatedly at night in a very distressed state. Her parents had adopted the practice of letting her go to sleep downstairs in their arms and then allowing her to sleep in their own bed every night. She woke every hour or two and needed much comforting before she settled back to sleep again each time. Her sleep was said to be restless and she snored most nights. Brief episodes of stiffening during sleep were also reported by her parents without any obvious relationship to the other nocturnal events.

She did not actually sleep during the day, but her behaviour was described as generally difficult. Her total sleep time per 24-hour period was typically about 7 hours compared with the average 11 to 12 hours for other children of her age. Treatment had consisted of baclofen for her spasticity. Chloral-containing compounds had been used for short periods but without any improvement in her sleep. Antiepileptic medication had not been used because her daytime seizures (described as episodes of unresponsiveness for up to 5 minutes' duration) were thought to be infrequent. There was a record of a single generalized tonic clonic seizure.

Comment: This case illustrates the need for wide-ranging assessments in such multiply disabled children. Physical factors which could have contributed to the child's severely limited and disrupted sleep include upper airway obstruction in sleep, nocturnal seizures (tonic seizures in particular may not be recognized as such) and discomfort in bed with difficulty changing position (possibly making respiratory problems worse). Parenting practices also needed to be modified. In particular, the child's dependence on her parents' presence and considerable attention at bedtime needed to be changed. Further assessment demonstrated that sleep-related breathing problems, discomfort at night and nocturnal seizures did not seem to be significant factors.

With persistence, it was possible to improve her settling and night-waking problems by means of the psychological approaches described in chapter 4. This was associated with some improvement in her behaviour, but further attempts to modify the way her parents handled her daytime behaviour difficulties were considered necessary.

Psychiatric disorder

The close connection between acute and chronic physical conditions and sleep disturbance is echoed in the many forms of acute and chronic psychological disorder (Stores, 1996). High rates of sleep disorder of various types are consistently described in child psychiatric groups compared with other children (Salzarulo & Chevalier, 1983; Simonds & Parraga, 1984; Sadeh et al., 1995).

The ways in which sleep disturbance and psychiatric disorders are linked are likely to be many and varied, including the possibility that both have a common origin. The 'chicken-and-egg' problem arises constantly: is the sleep disturbance one aspect of a psychological problem or are the daytime psychological difficulties (at least partly) the result of unsatisfactory sleep? The question is far from academic because the answer will determine where the main treatment emphasis should lie, i.e. on attempting to improve the child's daytime psychological difficulties (in the expectation that, if successful, this will automatically improve sleep) or on focused attempts to improve sleep itself. The causal relationship may become clear if, by means of careful history taking, the sequence of events can be identified, but this may well be difficult. In these circumstances, a therapeutic trial of one approach or the other is appropriate or, if this orderly procedure is not feasible, both may be attempted simultaneously. Even when daytime psychological difficulties cannot be wholly attributed to coexisting sleep problems, it is likely that successful attempts to improve sleep will be followed by less psychological disturbance during the day.

It should not be assumed that disturbed daytime behaviour is a barrier to the success of a behavioural programme for a sleep disorder; success in a relatively short period of time is possible even in severely learning disabled children with very difficult, so-called 'challenging' (i.e. very difficult) behaviour (Wiggs & Stores, 1998).

CASE: A 6-year-old boy with global developmental delay and epilepsy had both severe settling difficulties and daytime challenging behaviour. As bedtime approached he would become very agitated and would refuse to go to bed, screaming and coming back downstairs if his parents managed to get him to bed. Distressing struggles between the child and his mother lasted for up to an hour each night. Daytime tantrums and generally difficult behaviour were an additional source of distress. The family's general way of life was quite chaotic. In particular, his parents did not handle him consistently, often making threats which were never carried out.

A treatment programme was devised which initially involved trying to establish a pleasant bedtime routine. This was timed to coincide with the time he usually fell asleep (later than the time that the parents had been trying to get him to bed). Consequently, he was able to spend the evening with his parents (without any arguments) and, by the time the routine started, he was already sleepy. Mother then took him upstairs and stayed with him until he settled to sleep quite quickly. It was considered that the child no longer associated bedtime with upset and distress and had learned that the routine led to him going to his bedroom with his mother. Once he had accepted this and was falling asleep within 10 minutes of getting into bed, his mother began to leave the room for increasingly longer periods until he was able to settle to sleep by himself. The routine, and his bedtime, were then gradually brought forward by 10–15 minutes every few nights until a more appropriate bedtime was reached.

Comment: The parents still had difficulty managing the boy's daytime behaviour but, having been able to improve his settling problems in a systematic fashion, they felt more confident that his other behavioural problems could also be improved. (Psychological approaches to sleeplessness are discussed in chapter 4.)

Significant sleep disturbance has been reported in many types of psychiatric disorder.

- Difficulty getting to sleep, broken sleep, nightmares and night terrors are well-known problems in *anxious children* including those with *panic attacks* in whom night-time panic attacks can occur (Garland, 1995). Similar sleep disorders are described in *post-traumatic stress disorder* (PTSD) (Perrin et al., 2000) including children who have been abused (Glod et al., 1997) or subjected to the many other possible forms of stress or trauma, for example from a distressing change of school to involvement in a natural disaster (Sadeh, 1996). The sleep disturbance may persist for years, as in the case of burn injury (Kravitz et al., 1993).

Generalizations about the many types of trauma are limited in value and each type is best considered separately for both clinical and research purposes. The occurrence of some is obvious; others, in particular sexual abuse, may be covert. The possibility of concealed psychological trauma should be considered if a child is inexplicably afraid of sleep, being in bed or the dark, or has frequent disturbing parasomnias for no apparent reason (Sadeh et al., 1995).

Treatment of the sleep disturbance has been reported to improve the emotional state of children traumatized, for example, by burns (Roberts & Gordon, 1979), road traffic accident (Palace & Johnston, 1989) or sexual abuse (Dahl, 1996a). However, further research is needed to evaluate the therapeutic contribution of specific treatment for the sleep disturbance as part of overall care.

- Problems falling asleep and staying asleep is a main complaint of children and adolescents with severe *depressive disorders*, but about 25% report being excessively sleepy during the day (Ryan et al., 1987) possibly because of sleep onset difficulties (Dahl et al., 1996) and/or poor quality sleep (Sadeh et al., 1995). Considering that the major adverse effect of sleep deprivation appears to be mood change (Pilcher & Huffcutt, 1996), persistently disturbed sleep is likely to make depressive symptoms worse. For this reason, both the mood disorder of depressed people and their sleep disturbance should be treated specifically, and attention paid to good sleep hygiene. There have been inconsistent reports about the presence in young patients of the sleep-stage abnormalities (especially those concerning REM sleep and, in particular, shortened REM latency) which have been described as biological markers in some form of severe adult depression (Dahl & Puig-Antich, 1990).

  Seasonal affective disorder (SAD) is now recognized in children. The details of its presentation at this age remain to be clarified but include sleep disturbance in winter months in the form of sleeplessness or excessive sleepiness (Glod & Baidsen, 1999).

  The close relationship between sleep processes and mood, and physiological similarities between some forms of depression in adults and adolescents are suggested by the effectiveness in both of sleep deprivation in certain cases (Wirz-Justice & Van den Hoofdakker, 1999).

- Parents of children diagnosed as having *Attention Deficit Hyperactivity Disorder* (*ADHD*) report sleep problems very frequently, possibly more than in other child psychiatric groups (Chervin et al., 1997). The relationships between ADHD and sleep need to be clarified. ADHD is a general term covering different types of syndrome, and comorbidity (especially conduct disorder and oppositional behaviours) is common (Corkum et al., 1998). The limited number of studies in which sleep physiology has been examined in ADHD children has not always confirmed parental complaints. The various clinical and methodological reasons for this discrepancy have been discussed by Ball and Koloian (1995).

Sometimes ADHD symptoms have been attributed to definitive sleep disorders (e.g. obstructive sleep apnoea (OSA), periodic limb movements in sleep, circadian sleep–wake cycle disorders) in which the quality of the child's sleep is considered to be impaired or its duration shortened. ADHD symptoms are said to have improved with treatment of the sleep disorder (Dahl, 1996a). Where ADHD symptoms can be attributed to nonsleep factors, sleep disruption is likely to worsen the child's behaviour and, therefore, merits treatment in its own right. The best approach is likely to be behavioural, but the successful use of clonidine in otherwise difficult cases has been reported (Prince et al., 1996) although concerns have been expressed about the safety of combining clonidine with stimulant drugs (Poppwer, 1995).

Stimulant medications for ADHD symptoms are capable of producing physiological signs of disturbed sleep, and some reports suggest that sleep problems are associated clinically with their use (Stein, 1999). It is common practice to avoid administering them later in the day but, overall, the clinical significance of the reported effects of stimulant drugs on sleep physiology is debatable and some children may benefit from a later dose because it improves behaviour at bedtime (Chatoor et al., 1983). The need for further systematic research to clarify the relationships between ADHD and sleep disturbance have been emphasized by Corkum et al. (1998) and by Ball & Koloian (1995).

• There are many other psychiatric disorders in childhood and adolescence in which sleep disturbance is said to be a common complaint. *Autism* is a prominent example. The various sleep disorders described in autistic children include circadian sleep–wake cycle disorders (Stores & Wiggs, 1998a), the origin of which may reflect entrainment difficulties caused by impaired perception of social cues, or abnormal melatonin patterns (Patzold et al., 1998). The relationships between sleep disturbance and the *chronic fatigue syndrome* are complex and ill-defined (Stores, 1999b); sometimes a primary sleep disorder can be identified. Frequent awakenings, not obviously attributable to daytime inactivity, have been described in teenagers with this condition, suggesting that daytime symptoms might, at least partly, be explained by poor sleep quality (Stores et al., 1998b). It is important to consider the possibility that the chronic fatigue symptoms are the result of a sleep disorder.

CASE: Because of constant complaints of tiredness and disinterest in both school work and social activities over the past 2 years, a 16-year-old girl had been diagnosed by her psychiatrist as suffering from the chronic fatigue syndrome with depressive features. Her disinclination to get up in the morning had led to poor attendance at school and, following a 3-month period off school completely, she had been provided with home tuition for a few hours each week.

There was no obvious explanation for the onset of her symptoms. Physical examination and basic investigations were normal. A programme of graded increases in her physical activities was planned in the hope of an eventual return to school.

However, a new member of the psychiatric team, with some experience of working in a sleep disorders clinic, enquired about the patient's sleep pattern which had not been considered in any detail before. This revealed that for at least 2 years she had increasing difficulty getting to sleep at night sometimes not sleeping until 4 a.m. having gone to bed about 10 p.m. Before going to sleep, she was in the habit of reading or watching television in her bedroom or lying in bed wishing she could get to sleep. On weekdays, her mother had tried to rouse her at 8 a.m. to go to school but often she would go back to sleep until near midday. Except for the home tutor's brief visits, she spent the rest of the day by herself at home, which she found boring. Often she had an afternoon nap. At weekends she usually stayed in bed until early afternoon. There was no evidence of drug or alcohol abuse and she took caffeine-containing drinks only in moderation. There was no family history of significance.

In the light of this new information, and following consultation with the sleep disorders service, delayed sleep phase syndrome of uncertain origin was diagnosed and treatment, aimed at retiming her sleep phase, was started (see chapter 5). Explanation that this sleep disorder was likely to be the cause of her daytime symptoms was readily accepted by the family and the treatment programme was completed successfully, with an early return to school and improvement in her mood and social activities.

Comment: The importance of taking a sleep history as a routine is illustrated in this case, and also the need to consider that a primary sleep disorder might underlie psychiatric symptoms. The prompt response to treatment was gratifying but is not always achieved when the situation has become complicated by the secondary effects of the sleep disorder (such as prolonged absence from school) which are likely if recognition of the sleep disorder is delayed.

- Other psychiatric conditions where the nature of the sleep disturbance needs further investigation (see Stores, 1996 for references) include *substance abuse* (including withdrawal), *obsessive–compulsive disorder* (poor-quality sleep), *Tourette syndrome* (sleeplessness and parasomnias), *Asperger's syndrome* (hypersomnia), *eating disorders* (Benca & Casper, 2000) and *conduct disorders.* Occasionally in *Munchausen syndrome by proxy* parents complain about their child's sleep (Griffith & Slovik, 1989).
- The effects of *psychotropic medications* on sleep have been studied almost exclusively in adults, but a number of them used in children and adolescents are known to have adverse effects, namely sleeplessness or daytime sedation. Types of medication implicated in this way are psychostimulants, the various types of antidepressants or mood stabilizers, alpha agonists (e.g. clonidine), benzodiazepines and other types of anxiolytic drug, and neuroleptics (Mindell et al., 1999).

There is some evidence that in adults certain forms of psychotropic medication can induce other more specific sleep disorders. Examples are sleepwalking provoked by lithium, usually combined with neuroleptic drugs (Landry et al., 1999) or sedative–hypnotic drugs (Mendelson, 1994), and REM Sleep Behaviour Disorder induced by various psychotropic drugs (Sforza et al., 1997). In the absence of detailed information on the likelihood of these effects in young patients, at least an awareness of such possibilities is appropriate.

It is clear that a knowledge of sleep disturbance and its effects is essential for anyone working in paediatrics and also in child and adolescent psychiatry (including liaison work with paediatrics). This becomes even more obvious when the following effects of persistent sleep disturbance on psychological and physical development are considered.

Effects on development of persistent sleep disturbance

The serious concerns expressed by Dukes in 1905 stressed various physical consequences of inadequate sleep in young children, some of which are fanciful at first sight, in particular 'diminished growth of the brain and slight fainting attacks resembling epilepsy'. But the other effects that he suggested are not that far removed from evidence collected in more recent times about the adverse effects of severe sleep disturbance. 'Lowered vitality', 'apathy', 'bloodlessness' (in the figurative sense) all anticipate the evidence of impaired performance which has been linked with insufficient or poor-quality sleep. Diminished growth of body or failure to thrive has been linked with early onset obstructive sleep apnoea (OSA) and slow-wave sleep abnormalities in children. As will be mentioned later, there are indications that severe sleep disturbance can affect immune systems ('easy prey to disease').

Cognitive function and educational performance

There is extensive clinical and experimental evidence that sustained sleep disturbance can have serious adverse psychological effects in adults (Bonnet, 2000).

Experimental studies of *total sleep loss* demonstrate a progressive deterioration in cognitive function, mood and behaviour related to length of sleep loss. However, the nature and extent of these effects are influenced by the individual's motivation, personality and usual sleep requirements, as well as timing of the task in relation to the circadian sleep–wake cycle. Physical factors in the environment, such as noise or other distracting stimuli, are also important.

Some of these factors are also likely to explain individual differences in the effect of *partial sleep deprivation* which is much more common at any age than total sleep loss. Memory, attention and visuospatial abilities have been shown to be affected, especially sustained attention (vigilance), and possibly tasks requiring creative rather than purely logical thinking (Horne, 1988). It has been calculated that the average level of functioning of sleep-deprived adults is equivalent to only the 9th percentile of nonsleep-deprived subjects (Pilcher & Huffcutt, 1996).

In keeping with these experimental findings of impaired function, there are reports of impaired performance and increased accident rates in various occupational groups prone to persistent sleep disturbance (Dinges, 1995). There are also neuropsychological studies of patients (including children) with obstructive sleep apnoea whose sleepiness affects their cognitive function and mood which improve if the sleepiness is corrected (Engleman & Joffe, 1999). There have been similar reports concerning narcolepsy (Kashden et al., 1996).

These findings come very largely from studies of adults, but there is no reason, in principle, why comparable effects of chronic sleep deprivation should not occur in children and adolescents. Indeed, a number of recent reports suggest that this is so.

The very limited degree of experimental sleep deprivation that is ethically permissible in young subjects has been shown to result in objectively demonstrated increased daytime sleepiness (Ishihara, 1999), impaired psychomotor function and (possibly more so) verbal creativity and abstract thinking (Randazzo et al., 1998). Wolfson & Carskadon (1998) have pointed out the consistency with which their own and other studies have demonstrated that sleep loss in adolescents is associated with daytime sleepiness and impaired performance at school. They consider that this is probably a problem in most young people of that age in the USA, although high rates of such difficulties have been reported in various other countries such as The Netherlands (Meijer et al., 2000). The sleep loss, which tends to increase across the teenage years, results from late bedtimes and sometimes early starting times at school. Other reports have linked earlier bedtimes and more sleep with better academic attainment (see Wolfson & Carskadon, 1998).

Of the various clinical conditions mentioned earlier, upper-airway obstruction (usually by enlarged tonsils and adenoids) has been associated with children's poor academic performance and other psychological deficits, with improvement following adenotonsillectomy (Gozal, 1998). Adverse effects of nocturnal asthma appear to include impairment of some aspects of memory which recovers in association with impaired asthma control and a reduction in physiological sleep disruption (Stores et al., 1998c).

How long it takes for the adverse cognitive and other consequences of sleep loss to be reversed when satisfactory sleep is restored is not clear, certainly in children. In adults, clinical and polysomnographic recovery from short periods of sleep disturbance have been shown to occur after much less sleep than that originally lost, for example after 1–2 nights following several nights of sleep loss. There are indications that sleep physiology takes longer to return to normal in children than in adults, i.e. the usual rebound increase of SWS, followed by REM sleep, extending over several nights (Carskadon & Dement, 1981).

Emotional state and behaviour

A number of the studies just mentioned demonstrate that the adverse effects of persistent sleep disturbance are not confined to cognitive function but influence other aspects of psychological well-being. In fact, mood and behaviour may well be more affected than anything else (Pilcher & Huffcutt, 1996). The more usual general effects reported in adults are irritability and even aggression, depressed mood and complaints of fatigue or other physical symptoms such as aches and pains or gastrointestinal upset. More dramatic effects of prolonged and severe sleep disturbance in adults include disorientation, illusions, hallucinatory and persecutory ideas. Inappropriate behaviour with impaired awareness ('automatic behaviour') caused by frequent microsleeps is another possibility that is easily mistaken for psychiatric disorder.

One of the main differences between sleep disorders in adults and children is that sleepiness usually causes a reduction in activity in adults, but the opposite can occur in young children whose activity levels may be increased. As stated earlier, sleep disturbance at this age can produce a combination of overactivity, impulsiveness and poor concentration, together with irritability or other behavioural difficulties characteristic of ADHD.

The question of the direction of causal relationships is ever-present and is highlighted in the relationships between sleep disturbance and psychiatric disorder, notably those characterized by depression, anxiety or fatigue. It also applies to reports concerning children in the general population. For example, young schoolchildren who are sleepy are described as coping with difficulties less well and having more behaviour problems than other children (Wolfson & Carskadon, 1998; Lavigne et al., 1999). The evidence (described by the same authors) for sleep disturbance being the primary cause (or at least a major contributory factor) to the depressed mood, behavioural disturbance and academic difficulties of adolescents seems particularly compelling.

In addition to relatively direct ways in which psychological problems may result from sleep disturbance, a child's emotional state may be affected *indirectly* by the distress caused by aspects of his sleep disorder.

• For various reasons, bedtime can be an upsetting time. It may be associated with tension and confrontation between the child and his parents, punishment or other unpleasant experiences including fear of the dark, frightening sleep phenomena (such as hypnagogic hallucinations) or it may be associated with inability to sleep because of anxieties about daytime events.

• Sleep problems such as sleepwalking or snoring may be embarrassing, especially if they occur away from home. Some children react by denying the problem, or by becoming depressed or aggressive.

- Emotional development and behaviour may also be harmed by the effect of the child's sleep disturbance on other members of the family, especially parents. Depending on the nature of the sleep disturbance, parents (and sometimes siblings) may themselves suffer the effects of sleep deprivation. Alternatively, parents may be distressed if they misperceive the child's sleep problem as evidence of a serious underlying condition, as often happens with the more dramatic forms of sleepwalking or headbanging. The emotional climate within the family can be further affected if parents disagree about the best way to deal with the child's sleep problem or if the advice given is inconsistent or ineffective. The situation is also not helped if there are long delays before a correct diagnosis is made.

Depending on the circumstances, the consequences for parenting and family function can be very serious. Mothers of children with a learning disability and severe sleep problem have been described as more irritable, concerned about their own health and less affectionate towards their children (with greater use of physical punishment) than mothers of such children without sleep problems (Quine, 1992). There have also been suggestions that marital discord and separation, and even physical abuse of children, may result (Chavin & Tinson, 1980).

Clearly, it is essential to identify families in which these particularly unfortunate consequences are likely to occur and to intervene at an early stage. Psychosocial disadvantage and parental psychiatric disorder are likely warning signs. Prevention and treatment of such problems have received little attention, but preliminary findings suggest that treatment of a child's sleep problem can improve the mother's mental state, confidence in her own parenting ability and her relationships with her child, and also the child's behaviour (Wolfson et al., 1992; Quine, 1992; Minde et al., 1994).

Physical development

Impairment of physical growth can be associated with sleep disturbance (Carroll & Loughlin, 1995c). This and failure to thrive are recognized consequences of childhood OSA. The mechanisms involved are unclear. Growth hormone deficiency is not obviously the explanation. For example, children with OSA do not have a reduction in SWS with which growth hormone release is linked, and normal growth hormone levels have been described in some children with OSA and short stature. Other factors such as eating or sleeping difficulties may play their part. On the other hand, it has been suggested that 'psychosocial dwarfism' is the result of growth hormone abnormalities linked to sleep physiology (Taylor & Brooks, 1986).

There is also increasing interest in the interrelationships of sleep and immune systems and their implications for both physical and psychological well-being (Moldofsky & Dickstein, 1999).

Sleep disorders in child healthcare

Despite the relative neglect of sleep disorders medicine in children and adolescents, and the need for further research, there is clearly enough already known that is of central importance to clinical practice in paediatrics, child psychiatry and the allied disciplines concerned with child health and welfare.

Restated briefly, the argument in favour of sleep disorders medicine being viewed as a fundamental part of practice in these specialties and disciplines are as follows:

- *Sleep problems are common* in the general population, and particularly so in children with physical and psychiatric disorders including learning disability.
- The *consequences of persistent and severe sleep disturbance are likely to be serious* in their effects on mood, behaviour and cognitive function, and sometimes physical development, as well as on the family as a whole.
- In some instances, *sleep disturbance may be the primary cause of psychological or physical disorder* rather than a complication of an underlying condition.
- Sleep disturbance may be an *early-warning sign* of an impending, more obvious psychological or physical disorder. This has been particularly suggested for severe depressive or other major psychiatric disorders in adults (Ford & Kamerow, 1989). The same possibility should be considered in children and adolescents. Early vigorous treatment of the sleep disturbance may prevent the development or worsening of a psychological disturbance, or limit its duration.
- If the nature and range of sleep disorders are not appreciated, they *can be mistaken for a primarily psychological problem*. A main example of this is pathological sleepiness (chapter 5).
- Especially with early recognition of the presence of a sleep disorder, and its accurate diagnosis, *effective treatment should be possible* to the immediate and long-term benefit of the child and his family.
- Failure to deal effectively with childhood sleep disturbance may result in *sleep problems and their consequences extending into adult life* (Philip & Guilleminault, 1996).

Given these compelling reasons for considering sleep medicine to be fundamentally important, it is necessary to improve professional teaching and training as well as general awareness of this neglected area of clinical practice. The purpose of the following chapters is to help to achieve this by describing in an essentially clinical way, for those who have not taken a special interest in the topic, the modern approach to sleep disorders and their treatment in children and adolescents.

3

Basic aspects of sleep and its disorders

General aspects of normal sleep

In this section, following some general points about the nature and functions of sleep, the main aspects of normal sleep in adults will be described as the basis for a comparison of children's sleep. The emphasis is placed on findings of clinical significance. More detailed information can be found in, for example, the textbook of adult sleep disorders medicine by Kryger et al. (2000).

The nature of sleep

Sleep is a reversible state of reduced awareness of, and responsiveness to the environment. Usually it occurs when lying down, quietly, with little movement.

Sleep is physiologically distinct from other states of relative inactivity such as coma, stupor or hibernation. Within sleep two physiologically distinct states have been defined: Non-Rapid Eye Movement (NREM) sleep and REM sleep.

Both these forms of sleep are active processes. Wakefulness is maintained by cortical noradrenaline, dopamine and acetylcholine release from terminals of brainstem neurones. Activity in the ascending reticular activating system must diminish for sleep to occur. In addition, however, NREM sleep depends on activity in the basal forebrain systems especially, while mechanisms in the pons are primarily responsible for the control of REM sleep. Serotonin and gamma-aminobutyric acid (GABA) neurones are involved in NREM sleep; acetylcholine is essentially involved in the generation of REM sleep. Recent advances in functional neuroimaging are starting to provide further insights into the brain mechanisms of human sleep (Maquet, 1999).

There is no single sleep-promoting substance within the nervous system. Many substances have been implicated, including various neuropeptides, each of which, however, appears to have specific effects on sleep regulation (Steiger & Holsboer, 1997).

The functions of sleep

The various theories about the function of sleep have emphasized physical and psychological restoration and recovery, energy conservation, memory consolidation, discharge of emotions, brain growth and other biological functions including maintenance of immune systems. No one theory accounts for all the complexities of sleep in different species and at different stages of development, and it seems likely that sleep serves multiple purposes (Rechtschaffen, 1998).

The most obvious fact about sleep is that persistent disturbance causes psychological and sometimes physical impairment. Animals totally deprived of sleep for very long periods die following loss of temperature regulation and multiple system failure. As described earlier, the adverse effects of chronic partial sleep deprivation on mood, behaviour and cognitive function can be substantial.

The physiological changes associated with sleep disturbance (i.e. aspects of electroencephalography (EEG), autonomic, biochemical and endocrine function) that have been studied in humans mainly in relation to experimental sleep loss, have shown either no change or the changes have reversed fairly promptly when sleep patterns have returned to normal. At present it is difficult to define the apparently more subtle physiological changes which underly the various neuropsychological deficits and psychiatric disturbances.

Sleep stages

A major milestone in the history of sleep research was the distinction made between REM and NREM sleep (Aserinsky & Kleitman, 1953). Conventionally, standardized criteria (Rechtschaffen & Kales, 1968) are used to identify the different sleep stages according to their characteristic physiological features, especially in the EEG, electro-oculogram (EOG) and electromyogram (EMG). The main features of the different stages are shown in Table 1.

- *NREM sleep* is divided into 4 stages of increasing depth.

  Stage 1 occurs at sleep onset or following arousal from another stage of sleep. The EEG is low voltage with mixed frequencies and reduced alpha activity compared with the awake state. The EEG contains vertex sharp waves and slow rolling eye movements are seen. This stage represents 4–5% of the main sleep period.

  Stage 2 contains more slow activity, and sleep spindles and K complexes are seen. It accounts for 45–55% of overnight sleep.

  Stage 3 (4–6% of total sleep time) contains yet more slow EEG activity.

  Stage 4 is characterized by the most slow activity and constitutes 12–15% of sleep. The combination of stages 3 and 4 is called *slow wave sleep* (*SWS*) or *delta sleep*. This is considered to be the deepest form of sleep from which awakening is particularly difficult.

Table 1. Sleep stages: main features

Non-Rapid Eye Movement (NREM) sleep		
Stage 1	Mixed EEG frequencies	4–5% of main sleep period
	Reduced alpha activity	
	Vertex sharp waves	
	Slow rolling eye movements	
Stage 2	More slow EEG activity	45–55%
	Sleep spindles	
	K complexes	
Stage 3	Yet more slow EEG activity	4–6%
Stage 4	Predominantly slow activity	12–15%
Stages 3 & 4 referred to as slow wave sleep (SWS), delta sleep or deep sleep.		
Rapid Eye Movement (REM) sleep		
	Low voltage, mixed frequency nonalpha rhythm EEG	20–25%
	Spontaneous rapid eye movements	
	Skeletal muscle virtually paralysed	
	Variable heart rate, blood pressure and respiration	
	Body temperature regulation impaired	
	Penile and clitoral tumescence	
Brain metabolism at its highest in REM sleep		
Most dreaming occurs in REM sleep		

- *REM sleep* is physiologically very different from NREM sleep. Brain metabolism is highest in this stage of sleep with a low voltage, mixed frequency, nonalpha rhythm EEG. Spontaneous rapid eye movements are seen and EMG activity is virtually absent in the skeletal musculature. REM sleep has been called 'paradoxical sleep' because of the near absence of muscle tone despite the high levels of brain activity. Heart rate, blood pressure and respiration are all variable, body temperature regulation ceases temporarily, and penile and clitoral tumescence occurs. REM sleep usually takes up 20–25% of total sleep time.
  Most dreaming occurs in REM sleep.

Sleep architecture

NREM and REM sleep alternate cyclically throughout the night, starting with a period of NREM sleep lasting about 80 minutes followed by about 10 minutes of REM sleep. This 90 minutes 'sleep cycle' is repeated 3–6 times each night. Each REM period typically ends with a brief arousal or transition into light NREM sleep.

In successive cycles, the amount of NREM sleep decreases and the amount of

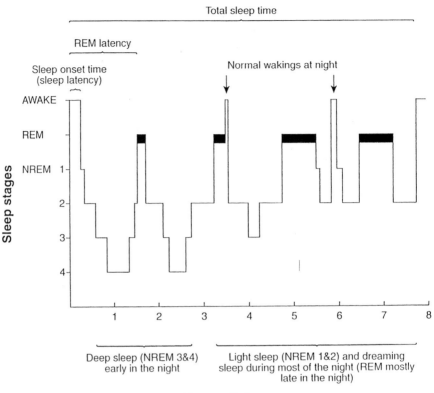

Hours of sleep

Figure 1   Hypnogram of healthy young adult.

REM sleep increases. SWS is usually confined to the first two sleep cycles. The diagrammatic representation of overnight sleep architecture is known as a '*hypnogram*', a simplified form of which is shown in Figure 1.

Sleep microstructure and sleep fragmentation

The conventional sleep staging just described is concerned with the 'macrostructure' of sleep, but there is increasing interest in the microstructural disruption of sleep by frequent, brief arousals (seen mainly as changes in the EEG) lasting a matter of seconds without obvious clinical accompaniments. This subtle disruption of sleep continuity is overlooked by conventional sleep staging and can occur without any significant reduction in total sleep time or conventional sleep stages. It has been associated with daytime sleepiness and impairment of performance, mood and behaviour (Roth et al., 1994).

The limited normative data available from healthy subjects suggest that, between the teenage years and old age, brief arousals are a basic physiological aspect of sleep

(Boselli et al., 1998). Their number (but not their duration) increases steadily with age, but the borderline between normal and abnormal rates of arousals is ill-defined at present. A high rate of brief arousals is known to occur in response to arousing stimuli in certain pathological conditions during sleep such as apnoea, leg movements and pain. In other cases the cause is not obvious. Like other interruptions to night-time sleep, such arousals tend to increase in the elderly.

The term *fragmentation* of sleep refers to the frequent occurrence of brief arousals and/or other frequent interruptions of sleep including those involving awakenings. These effects on *sleep continuity* are an important undermining influence on the restorative *quality of sleep*, often more so than other changes in sleep, although the combination of fragmented sleep and partial sleep loss is particularly harmful (Gillberg, 1995). Wider aspects of sleep microstructure, such as the 'cyclic alternating pattern' (CAP) of arousal level during sleep, including its possible relevance to various disorders of sleep, have been discussed by Terzano and Parrino (2000).

Circadian sleep–wake rhythms

The timing of sleep (but not its amount) is regulated by a circadian clock in the suprachiasmatic nucleus (SCN) of the hypothalamus. Without environmental cues to time of day (or '*zeitgebers*', literally 'time givers'), the duration of the endogenous 'free running' sleep–wake cycle in humans has generally been considered to be about 25 hours, although recent reports have cast some doubt on this and suggest that the intrinsic circadian pacemaker is close to 24 hours in human adults, consistent with other species (Czeisler et al., 1999). From a very early age, the individual's sleep–wake rhythm has to synchronize with the 24-hour day–night cycle. The main zeitgeber by which this is achieved ('*entrainment*') is light, but social cues (such as mealtimes and social activities) are also important as well as ambient temperature or noise level, and internal body signals such as hunger, temperature and hormonal changes.

The SCN also controls other biological rhythms including body temperature and cortisol production with which the sleep–wake rhythm is normally synchronized. Growth hormone, in contrast, is locked to the sleep–wake cycle and is released with the onset of SWS, whatever its timing.

The hormone *melatonin* is related to the light–dark cycle rather than the sleep–wake cycle (Zhdanova, 2000). It is mainly produced in the pineal gland from where it is secreted during darkness ('the hormone of darkness') and suppressed by exposure to bright light. It influences circadian rhythms via the SCN pacemaker which, in turn, regulates melatonin secretion by relaying light information to the pineal gland. In recent years, it has achieved popularity as a sleep promoting agent although its use remains contentious (see later in this chapter).

The tendency to sleep displays an ultradian pattern in which sleepiness is greater in the early hours of the morning and again, to a lesser extent, in the early afternoon (the '*postlunch dip*'). Fluctuations in performance reflect this pattern (Mitler & Miller, 1996). Performance errors in various occupations (and indeed the timing of deaths from various diseases) show this two-peak pattern of occurrence. Level of alertness is generally at its highest in the evening before the onset of sleepiness as bedtime approaches. This period has been called the '*forbidden zone*' when sleep is particularly difficult to attain (Lavie, 1986). However, individual differences are seen in the precise timing of this pattern. Even from an early age, some people wake early and are especially alert and active in the morning then tire in the evening and are soon asleep ('*morning types*' or '*larks*'). Others are at their best in the evening and find it particularly difficult to get up and function in the morning ('*evening types*' or '*owls*') (Horne & Ostberg, 1979). Although little studied, such differences are thought to exist in children from an early age (Ferber, 1987).

Sleep duration

Most young adults report sleeping 7 to 8 hours a night during the week and rather longer at weekends. However, individuals differ, some needing much more than this and others much less. Total sleep time decreases in the elderly to about 5–6 hours on average because sleep is less well maintained than at an earlier age.

Characteristic features of sleep in childhood and adolescence

Although sleep changes across the whole life span, the most profound alterations take place during childhood, many being complete as early as about 6 months of age. The general progression in early childhood is towards differentiation and organization of conventionally defined sleep states, shorter total time spent asleep, less SWS and longer sleep cycles. Details of normal sleep from the neonatal period to adolescence can be found in Kahn et al. (1996). The main differences between adults and children in the architecture of overnight sleep are listed in Table 2.

- The special nature of sleep in early infancy is reflected in a manual for scoring states of sleep and wakefulness in the newborn (Anders et al., 1971). Three basic sleep states are described in full-term infants: *active sleep* (comparable to adult REM sleep); *quiet sleep* (an immature form of NREM sleep); and *indeterminate* or *transitional sleep* (a mixture of the other two). Until about 6 months of age the first part of sleep consists of active sleep.
- The *circadian rhythms* of temperature, waking, melatonin output and then (at a somewhat later stage) sleeping are all capable of developing very rapidly, i.e. within the first weeks to months of life, under the influence of both light changes

Table 2. Architecture of children's overnight sleep compared with adults (see Figure 1)

Longer total sleep time depending on age (Table 3)
SWS particularly prominent in young children
Early reduction in proportion of REM sleep
Greater number of NREM/REM sleep cycles
Possible period of SWS before finally waking

Table 3. Average sleep duration at different ages

Full-term birth	16–18 hours
1 year	15 hours
2 years	13–14 hours
4 years	12 hours
10 years	8–10 hours
Mid adolescence	$8\frac{1}{2}$ hours
Later adolescence	7–8 hours

(especially sunlight) and regular social cues (McGraw et al., 1999).

- In the first 2–3 months of life, rhythmic *melatonin* secretion does not occur (Kennaway et al., 1992) but afterwards there is a rapid increase until peak nighttime levels between 1 and 3 years of age. Levels then decline, especially at the onset of puberty (Waldhauser et al., 1988) although individual differences are prominent (Cavallo, 1992). About the same time there is a change in the timing of melatonin secretion which is associated with a delay in the overnight sleep phase independent of psychosocial influences (Carskadon et al., 1997). After adolescence, levels decline only moderately until old age. Normative data for circulating melatonin are not well defined at any age.

- *Total sleep time* reduces from 16 to 18 hours a day in newborns to the 7–8 hours of adult life which is achieved by adolescence. Sleep is usually confined to night time by about 3 years of age. Table 3 shows the typical amounts of sleep taken at different ages in childhood and adolescence although, again, it is important to know that sleep requirements vary with the individual. In young children still taking naps, the total amount of sleep per 24 hours may be divided between night and day in different proportions from one child to another. The continuous decrease in total sleep time of 2 hours or more during adolescence is considered to be largely environmentally determined and generally disadvantageous (see chapter 5).

- *SWS* is particularly prominent in young children who sleep very soundly and are difficult to wake. It is suggested that, apart from other factors, this amount of

SWS predisposes children of that age to arousal disorders (such as sleepwalking and sleep terrors) which usually arise from this stage of sleep. Sleep disorders (such as OSA) which in adults cause a reduction in SWS do not have this effect. This might partly explain why extreme degrees of daytime sleepiness are not necessarily seen in children of this age with such disorders.

- Most children between about 5 years of age and puberty sleep particularly soundly and are very alert during the day. Various conditions which cause excessive daytime sleepiness in adults may not have this effect in children of this age because of their high level of alertness (although overnight sleep may become longer).

- In contrast, many adolescents are sleepy during the day. Their amount of SWS becomes proportionately less than at an earlier age, the timing of their sleep phase may be physiologically delayed and, with the onset of puberty, sleep requirements do not continue to decrease as they had steadily done so throughout earlier development. These physiological changes often combine with strong social influences to stay up late, especially at weekends, and possibly other pressures during the week to get up early. This is likely to produce unsatisfactory sleep–wake patterns, excessive sleepiness and various psychological problems during the day (chapter 5).

- The proportion of *REM* sleep declines from 50% or more of total sleep time in the newborn (more than this in premature babies) to 20–25% by 2 years of age. This figure remains fairly constant throughout the rest of life. The high level of REM sleep in very early life suggests a role in cerebral maturation, but at present its true significance remains unclear (Goodale, 1994).

- *NREM/REM sleep cycles* occur at intervals of 50–60 minutes in infants who often enter REM sleep at the start of their sleep period. This interval between sleep cycles continues until adolescence when the periodicity changes to 90–100 minutes which persists into adult life. The amounts of NREM and REM in each sleep cycle is about equal in early infancy; afterwards NREM sleep (especially SWS) predominates in the earlier cycles and REM sleep in the later cycles. Young children may have a period of SWS before finally waking in the morning.

- *Continuity of sleep* varies considerably during childhood. It was suggested earlier that the fragility of sleep in early infancy is possibly the result of the prominence of REM sleep. As just mentioned, sleep in childhood is generally sound, although (as at all other ages) awakenings during the night are normal but often not recalled unless there is difficulty returning to sleep. Normative data from sleep recordings at home show only a tendency for the number of awakenings to increase with age between 5 and 15 years (Stores et al., 1998a).

- *Fragmentation* of sleep by arousals has received little attention in children. However, norms have recently been compiled for children of school age (Stores

& Crawford, 2000) which will help the clinical significance of this feature in sleep disorders to be assessed.

- *Circadian sleep–wake rhythms* change considerably in early development. Full-term neonates show 3–4 hour sleep–wake cycles. Sleep periods have largely shifted to the night and wakefulness to daytime by 12 months, except for daytime napping.
- There is a gradual reduction in the number of *daytime naps* from between 4 and 6 in the newborn, 2–3 naps by about 6 months and then to 1 nap by about 1 year. After 3–4 months, naps do not usually last longer than about 2–2.5 hours altogether, and most children have stopped napping by 3–5 years of age, although a few continue until about 7 (Weissbluth, 1995a).
- The previously mentioned ultradian rhythms in sleepiness, the 'owls' and 'larks' distinction, and the notion of the 'forbidden zone' in the evening are important in children as well as adults.

Definition of sleep problems

What is considered a sleep problem varies considerably from one family to another. Sleep-related behaviours which are very worrying to some parents are of no concern to others. Conversely, parents may be complacent (or at least not seek help) when their child's sleep pattern should be altered in the interests of the child and possibly the family as a whole.

The influence of cross-cultural differences in child-rearing practices on children's sleep patterns can be striking. Lozoff (1995) has illustrated this for thumb sucking and use of 'attachment or transitional (comfort-giving) objects' to help the child to sleep, feeding practices (including how they affect the establishment of sleep–wake patterns in infants), and whether children should be encouraged to sleep alone or with their parents. Encouraging children to sleep alone is a relatively new practice in Western society. In the USA, major differences in this respect have been described between different ethnic and socioeconomic groups.

Within any one cultural or subcultural group, preferences and practices are likely to vary according to each family's circumstances (including its structure, cohesion and organization) as well as parents' commitments, personality and health. All these factors can influence parents' perception of their child's sleep habits and behaviours, and their ability and willingness to change the way they handle their child. Some of these influences require attention in their own right (maternal depression is an obvious example), but generally it is not appropriate to be prescriptive about the way the family should conduct itself. Criticism is likely to be resented and suggested changes resisted. Where change is considered desirable in the interests of the child and family, tactful persuasion is usually more productive.

Parents' attitudes to the child's sleep are also influenced by their own expectations and ideas of what is normal and, for a variety of reasons (including straightforward misinformation), these may be seriously mistaken. In such cases, parents can be reassured that what they perceive as a problem (e.g. regarding how long their child should sleep) is within the normal range. Sometimes mistaken views can be changed by providing correct information; in other cases, the origin of parents' distorted views of the child may be more complicated, such as a general antipathy to the child or an inability to cope with normal childhood behaviour.

Conversely, parents may not be concerned about the child's sleep when they should be. They may be unaware of the problem (e.g. where the child conceals his night-time fears) or indifferent, or mistaken in their view of the child's behaviour (which happens when pathologically sleepy states are misconstrued as laziness or boredom). A rather different reason for not seeking help can be a mistaken belief that the child's troublesome sleep pattern is irreversible or untreatable, as expressed by some parents of children with particularly severe sleep disturbance (Wiggs & Stores, 1998).

Ways in which sleep can be disturbed

Sleep can be disturbed in three basic ways: loss of sleep, poor quality sleep and inappropriate timing of the period of sleep. Combinations of all three are possible. Ideally, each aspect should be assessed.

- *Loss of sleep* rarely takes the form of *total loss*. The usual problem is *partial sleep deprivation*, i.e. a reduction in the total hours of sleep compared with the child's usual amount of sleep. This can be caused by going to bed late, or inability to get to sleep until late, combined with having to get up before enough sleep has been obtained. This failure to meet sleep requirements may also result from waking or being woken very early.

  Because of individual differences, shortage of sleep is best judged in relation to how long the child usually sleeps. Like many other biological variables, individual sleep requirements are distributed normally with some children needing much less and others much more than the average without there being any sleep pathology. However, the sleep loss problem may have lasted so long that the child's usual sleep pattern is misleading. It is useful, therefore, to know how long children of different ages usually sleep (see Table 3). If a given child's sleep is consistently less by, say, 1 hour or more than the average for his age (especially if there is evidence of underperformance or behavioural disturbance during the day) additional sleep may be beneficial.

  It has been debated whether partial sleep deprivation, and its own adverse effects on daytime performance and behaviour, are endemic in Western civilization. Some argue in favour of the notion of a 'national sleep debt' (Bonnet & Arand, 1995). Others dispute this idea (Harrison & Horne, 1995). The extent to which partial sleep deprivation affects young members of the community is unclear but, as described in the previous chapter, teenagers appear to be at particular risk. Some younger children seem to perform better and to feel better with extra time asleep even when they have shown no obvious signs of not sleeping long enough.

- There is also debate about what constitutes *poor quality sleep*, involving which aspect of sleep is most important restoratively. Arguments have been advanced for both slow wave sleep and REM sleep. For example, SWS is replenished first in recovery sleep following sleep deprivation; on the other hand, as described earlier, REM sleep is particularly prominent in the early phases of human development. More recently, emphasis has been placed by some on the first few NREM/REM cycles in the first two-thirds or so of overnight sleep ('core sleep') which contains most SWS and some REM sleep. The remaining part of sleep at night has been referred to as 'optional' with some evidence that at least some adults can learn to curtail it without serious consequences (Horne, 1991). How generally true this is for adults has not been established, and whether it applies at all to children is unknown.

It was mentioned earlier that *disturbance of the continuity of sleep* appears to particularly impair its quality (Bonnet, 2000). Frequent obvious awakenings are clearly disruptive but clinical and experimental evidence indicates that frequent brief arousals, without clinical accompaniment at the time, impair the restorative value of sleep. Obviously, information about these physiological events is not available in usual clinical practice, although, in cases where there is suspicion that impaired sleep quality of a more subtle kind might be affecting daytime learning and behaviour, it should be sought. More usually a cruder index of poor sleep quality has to be made in terms of reported or observed interruptions of sleep continuity by frequent awakenings, or possibly very restless sleep. However, 'restless sleep' is an ambiguous term with ill-defined physiological accompaniments. Sometimes it refers to gross general movements during sleep to various degrees; otherwise parents might use the term to describe noisy sleep, talking during sleep or interruptions of their child's sleep by various events including parasomnias (chapter 6).

- *Inappropriate timing of the sleep period* is also associated in adults with poor-quality sleep and psychological impairment when awake. Night shift-work is the obvious example (Akerstedt, 1998). The abnormal timing of sleep (in the increasing numbers of people involved in such work) is often associated with a reduction in the hours of sleep and also impaired sleep quality. Adjusting to the shift-work is often difficult, and various psychological and physical complaints develop. Work performance suffers, including the occurrence of an increased number of accidents.

Anecdotally, parental shift-work can affect children's sleep. Bedtime may be set to allow parents to spend time with their child before or after work. In addition, the domestic arrangements for child care while the parents are at work can disrupt the child's sleep–wake pattern (see also chapter 4).

In young people, a situation comparable to that in adults can develop if the timing and amount of sleep (and other activities) keep changing. This irregularity of the sleep–wake schedule, and also mistiming of the sleep phase as discussed in later chapters, are most commonly seen in adolescents, but may also occur in younger children if their parents do not establish consistent day and night-time routines.

Discussion of the effects of persistent sleep disturbance is generally not based on a particularly thorough assessment of sleep in terms of duration, quality and timing. The relative importance of these aspects of children's sleep has been studied only sporadically. For example, there are indications that, of the various groups of sleep problem encountered in children with Down syndrome, those in which there is a reduction in the duration and continuity of overnight sleep are particularly associated with psychological disturbance during the day (Stores, R. et al., 1998). Poor-quality sleep, characterized by frequent wakenings (both prolonged and brief), have been linked with depressed mood and cognitive and behavioural problems in children with asthma (Stores et al., 1998c). A similar association between reduced sleep quality and daytime underfunctioning has also been reported in children with apparently well-controlled asthma (Sadeh et al., 1998). By analogy with adult studies, poor quality sleep with fragmentation by brief arousals might be expected in children with OSA (in whom daytime psychological difficulties are common) although, curiously, absence of such fragmentation has been reported (Guilleminault et al., 1982).

Despite the limited amount of research on children, enough is known (supplemented by reasonable extrapolations from adult studies) to alert the clinician to ways in which both psychological and physical aspects of development might be affected by sleep disturbance of one type or another and particularly when different forms of disturbance are combined.

Identifying sleep disturbance

Some forms of sleep disturbance are obvious by any standards, including dramatic and worrying nighttime episodes, but parents who are sensitive to the possibility that their child's sleep is disturbed, and that his well-being is compromised as a result, may be unsure about what is acceptable and ask what they should look for in order to detect the problem.

- Bedtime struggles and demands for their attention during the night may be viewed by them as an inevitable part of child development, but they should at least be acquainted with the fact that these are problems for which help is available.
- Similarly, they should be alerted to the need for investigation if their child falls asleep repeatedly during the day beyond the age at which daytime napping is normal (usually 5 at the latest).
- The same applies if the child is particularly difficult to wake in the morning, or is especially irritable and unpleasant about being woken, as this suggests inadequate or poor-quality sleep. In contrast, waking spontaneously at the right time is reassuring. Especially in teenagers, difficulty getting up in the morning and going to sleep late should not be automatically viewed as adolescent 'awkwardness' (see chapter 5).
- Failure to get to sleep until well after going to bed (for which there are many possible explanations according to age of the child) needs to be corrected.
- Less obvious daytime signs of unsatisfactory sleep are poor concentration and memory, deterioration in school work, and irritable or otherwise difficult behaviour. Of course, there are often other explanations for these problems, but sleep loss or disruption should be considered as a possibility.
- It is useful to estimate the total time the child sleeps to see if it is very different from the norm for sleep duration at his age (Table 2). However, bearing in mind individual differences at any age, it is sometimes more useful to see if the child's daytime problems have been associated with an obvious reduction or other change in his sleep.
- If the child's sleep can be extended, it might be found that the difficulty getting up in the morning and the daytime difficulties improve.

Schemes for classifying sleep disorders

Sleep problems and sleep disorders

The starting-point for the clinician is the child's *sleep problem* (as described usually by his parents) which will be one (or more) of three basic types:

- difficulty getting to sleep or staying asleep;
- sleeping too much;
- disturbed episodes related to sleep.

The aim is to identify the specific *sleep disorder* (or underlying cause) from the many that can give rise to these problems. The distinction between the sleep problem and the explanation for it is essential. It is readily accepted that the complaint of breathlessness, for example, needs to be explained in terms of the underlying cause and treated accordingly. However, sleep problems are often considered only at the symptomatic level.

For example, as will be discussed in chapter 4, the common problem in young children of difficulty getting off to sleep can be the result of many different factors. These include failure on the part of parents to establish satisfactory bedtime behaviours, overstimulation of the child before or at bedtime, putting the child to bed too early, an environment that is not conducive to sleep, or negative feelings on the child's part about going to bed (such as fear of the dark or being left alone). In some cases, the child is not physiologically ready to sleep because his sleep phase has become delayed. Obviously, each of these explanations calls for a different solution to the bedtime settling problem. Some sleep disorders may cause more than one type of complaint and a child may have more than one sleep disorder.

There are a number of systems that are used for classifying sleep disorders.

DSM and ICD systems

Both these systems provide schemes for classifying a range of sleep disorders but they do so in different ways. *DSM-IV* allocates sleep disorders to three broad categories: primary sleep disorders, sleep disorders related to mental disorders, and other sleep disorders. In the *ICD-10* classification, sleep disorders are dispersed over various sections: mental disorders; diseases of the nervous system and sense organs; and symptoms, signs and ill-defined conditions.

The International Classification of Sleep Disorders

The recently revised International Classification of Sleep Disorders or ICSD-R (American Sleep Disorders Association, 1997) is a more comprehensive, logical, informative and up-to-date scheme than the DSM and ICSD systems. The 80 or more sleep disorders it describes are grouped as shown in Table 4.

- *Dyssomnias* are primary sleep disorders which cause either difficulty getting off to sleep or remaining asleep (insomnia or sleeplessness), or excessive sleepiness during the day. The dyssomnias are divided into *intrinsic sleep disorders* (originating from within the body), *extrinsic sleep disorders* (caused by external factors) and *circadian rhythm sleep disorders* (related to the timing of sleep within the 24-hour period).

- *Parasomnias* (disturbances which intrude into the sleep process) are subdivided according to the phase of sleep with which they are associated: *arousal disorders* (arising from NREM sleep); *sleep–wake transition disorders*, and *parasomnias usually associated with REM sleep. Other parasomnias* are those which do not fall into these three categories.

- *Sleep Disorders Associated with Mental, Neurological or other Medical Disorders*

Table 4. International classification of sleep disorders – revised (1997)

Dyssomnias
A   Intrinsic sleep disorders
B   Extrinsic sleep disorders
C   Circadian rhythm sleep disorders

Parasomnias
A   Arousal disorders
B   Sleep–wake transition disorders
C   Parasomnias usually associated with REM sleep
D   Other parasomnias

Sleep disorders associated with mental, neurological or other medical disorders
A   Associated with mental disorders
B   Associated with neurological disorders
C   Associated with other medical disorders

Proposed sleep disorders

are not primary sleep disorders but sleep related manifestations of psychiatric or medical conditions.

• Conditions which need further assessment before each can be convincingly seen as a disorder in their own right are called *Proposed Sleep Disorders*.

ICSD-R provides useful summaries of each sleep disorder including its main features, associated features and possible complications, course, predisposing factors, prevalence, age at onset, sex ratio, familial patterns, polysomnographic and other laboratory features, and differential diagnosis. Diagnostic, severity and duration criteria are also stated. By means of a 3-axis system, a patient's condition and treatment needs can be characterized in terms of the ICSD diagnosis of the sleep disorder, investigations performed and particular abnormalities demonstrated, and accompanying medical and psychiatric disorders. A glossary of basic terms and concepts is also provided (see end of this book).

For the most part, the structure of the ICSD will be followed in this book, with occasional modification as considered clinically appropriate.

Differences between sleep disorders in children and adults

Despite its good points overall, the ICSD-R is essentially adult-based and needs to be modified somewhat when used for children and adolescents. This is preferable to attempts to devise a separate system which would add to the risk of children's sleep disorders medicine being viewed as separate from its adult counterpart. Important considerations when using the ICSD for young patients are as follows.

Patterns of sleep behaviours and disorders in children

- Throughout childhood, *striking and often rapid changes* occur compared with the much longer time course of events in adult life. By the same token, the *range of sleep behaviours and disorders* in children is particularly wide.
- Some *sleep behaviours which are developmentally usual in children are abnormal in adults* and require investigation. Examples are repeated napping and wetting at night in very young children.
- Certain sleep disorders are seen *exclusively in children*, for example bedtime problems related to 'infantile colic'. Others, such as settling problems, head-banging and arousal disorders, occur *primarily in children*.
- *Dyssomnias caused by extrinsic factors* (mainly child rearing practices) are particularly common in early childhood. Those attributable to *circadian sleep–wake rhythm disorders* (especially the delayed sleep phase syndrome) can occur at all ages, but are considered to be commonplace in adolescents.
- Some *sleep disorders thought to be essentially adult conditions are now recognized in children*. Examples include obstructive sleep apnoea and REM sleep behaviour disorder.

A serious omission in the ICSD-R is any mention in the section concerned with mental, neurological and other medical disorders that sleep problems are commonly associated with learning disability.

Parenting factors

In adult sleep disorders, partners and other family members might be implicated or affected in various ways, but there is no real counterpart in adults to the pervading influence of parents in the origin, course and treatment of many children's sleep disorders. Even in basically physical sleep disorders, parenting factors are often important. Examples have already been given of the influence of parents in the definition, recognition and cause of children's sleep problems, as well as the possible serious effects of the child's sleep disturbance on parenting practices and competence. The importance of parents in the treatment of sleep disorders will become obvious later when the correction of parenting practices or attitudes is discussed (chapter 4).

The attitudes and practices of parents in relation to the children's sleep habit and patterns may be important in other ways.

- Especially in the early years, most children need their parents' help in coping with separating from them at night, and the potentially frightening experience of the dark or their own thoughts and fantasies. Infants need comfort from physical contact. Toddlers benefit from bedtime routines and by comforting objects, as well as by being helped to fall asleep without their parents' presence and attention. The ability of parents to provide such help depends on their personality and sensitivity, their circumstances and their own emotional state. Hopefully, older children and adolescents become increasingly independent.

- Much harm can be done (perhaps long-term) if, instead of encouraging in their child positive attitudes to sleeping, parents create negative associations such as confrontation, punishment, rejection or in extreme cases abuse.
- Some parents are motivated to maintain their child's sleep problem for reasons that may be difficult to influence. For example, the child's presence in the parental bed might be welcomed by one partner as a means of distancing him/herself from the other at night. Sometimes a parent encourages the child to sleep with them as a source of comfort unavailable in other forms.

Manifestations of sleep disorders

The *clinical features* of basically the same sleep disorder can be very different in children compared with adults.

- The point was made earlier that, whereas the overall behavioural effects of excessive sleepiness in adults is a reduction of physical and mental activity, its effects in young children can be increased activity with irritability, tantrums or other behavioural problems.
- OSA illustrates important differences (described in chapter 5) between children and adults, not only in the clinical manifestation of a particular sleep disorder but also in the underlying causes and the treatment required.
- Similarly (as also discussed in chapter 5) the early manifestation of narcolepsy in childhood may be very far removed from the classical narcolepsy syndrome usually described in adults.

The same sleep disorder may also show different *physiological features* according to age. Diagnostic criteria (e.g. for OSA and narcolepsy) derived from polysomnographic studies in adults do not necessarily apply in children and may well need to be modified.

Significance

The possible adverse effects on adults of persistent sleep disturbance were emphasized in the first two chapters. As also explained in chapter 2, there is no particular reason to suppose that such harmful effects are any less likely at earlier stages of development. Indeed, it might be expected that they are more serious.

In another way, the significance of sleep disorders can vary with age, including the underlying causes and the need for intervention beyond treatment of the sleep disorder itself. Sleepwalking and other arousal disorders (chapter 6) appear to be a good example. A general rule of thumb (subject to revision in the light of further much needed research) is that childhood parasomnias of this type are not usually associated with any underlying psychological or physical disorder, whereas the same type of sleep disturbance in adults may well indicate one or other form of mental disturbance (Ohayon et al., 1999) or organic pathology in the elderly (Kefauver & Guilleminault, 1994).

Treatment and prognosis

In general, a more optimistic view can be taken of children's sleep disorders compared with adults. Children's sleep patterns may be easily disturbed by environmental or other factors. By the same token, however, they may readily change back again compared with adults in whom the factors underlying the sleep problem may have become well established and complicated by secondary effects. That being so, it is often appropriate to sound a particularly optimistic note about response to treatment, providing that the treatment is based on accurate diagnosis, and that appropriate measures are likely to be implemented by parents in a committed and systematic way.

Assessment of sleep disorders

The means by which sleep disorders can be detected and assessed need to be modified for use with children because of developmental factors, the involvement of parents, and the various differences between children and adults regarding the clinical manifestations of sleep disorders and also diagnostic criteria.

To prevent sleep problems being overlooked, the following basic screening questions should be asked routinely as part of taking a history about any child, whatever the setting:
• Does the child have difficulty getting to sleep or staying asleep?
• Is he excessively sleepy during the day?
• Does he have any disturbing episodes at night?
A positive answer to any of these questions calls for a detailed sleep history.

Sleep history

The sleep history is the cornerstone of assessment. Obviously, parents are the usual source of information, but children themselves should be questioned if they are old enough. Any disparities between the accounts given by parents and the child will need to be explained. Observations by siblings and teachers can also be important.

Because traditional history-taking schedules pay little attention to sleep, detailed sleep-related enquiries should be added to the questions that are usually asked. The main aspects to be covered are as follows:
• Precise nature of the sleep complaint, its start, development and current pattern.

- Medical or psychological factors at the start of the sleep problem, or which might have precipitated or maintained it.
- Patterns of occurrence of the symptoms, including factors making them better or worse, weekdays compared with weekends or with holiday periods.
- Effects on mood, behaviour, school work, friendships, general activities and other family members.
- Past and present treatment for the sleep problem and their effects, including exact methods used, for how long and who was involved.

Detailed information is also needed about the following aspects:

- The child's *24-hour sleep–wake schedule* (Table 5), bearing in mind the possibility of variation from one day to another and differences between weekdays and weekends. The evening meal is a useful starting-point, followed by preparation for and timing of bedtime; time and process of getting to sleep; events during the night disturbing the continuity of sleep (including their nature and timing); what happens if the child wakens or is disturbed at night; time and ease of waking up and getting up (spontaneous or induced waking); level of alertness, mental state and behaviour during the day; daytime naps; mealtimes and other daytime activities.

  Especially in young children, the circumstances in which the child goes to sleep are particularly important in determining what he associates with going to sleep. As explained later, if these '*sleep associations*' are unpleasant, the prospect of bedtime and sleeping will produce resistance or cause distress. If going to sleep is associated with parental attention, this becomes an unwelcome prerequisite for the child to settle to sleep and also for getting back to sleep when he wakes in the night.

- The child's '*sleep rhythm*', i.e. the timing and duration of the overnight sleep phase and any daytime naps, and the *overall amount of sleep* each 24 hours. As mentioned previously, the *duration, continuity and timing of the child's sleep* are the most important aspects of sleep for daytime functioning.
- *Events that may be of particular diagnostic significance* (e.g. chronic noisy breathing, including snoring).
- '*Sleep hygiene*' (see Table 6), i.e. how far the sleeping environment is satisfactory and whether the organization of the child's day and general activities (especially leading up to bedtime) are conducive to sleeping well.

Compilation of a sleep history can be aided by the use of a screening *sleep–wake questionnaire*. These have not been well developed for use with children, but there are some which are general in their scope (e.g. those developed by Bruni et al., 1996 or by Owens et al., 2000). Others are directed to particular aspects such as sleep-disordered breathing (Chervin et al., 2000) or an adaptation of the Epworth Sleepiness Scale or ESS, a brief questionnaire about sleepiness in everyday

Table 5. Review of child's 24-hour sleep–wake pattern (modified according to child's age)

Evening

What time is the child's last meal?

What activities typically take place between then and getting ready for bed?

Does the child take any sleep medicine?

Going to bed

Who gets the child ready for bed and how? Is it always the same person and done in the same way?

Is there a bedtime routine? If so, what is the sequence of events? Does it include a wind-down period?

What time does he go to bed?

Is he put to bed awake or asleep?

Where and how does he fall asleep (own bed, parent's bed, downstairs, being rocked, nursed or fed, with or without a parent present?)

Does he need a bottle, dummy or special object to fall asleep or want someone else to sleep with?

Does he express fears about going to bed?

Does he have his own room?

Is the bedroom conducive to sleep or is it a place for entertainment or other arousing experiences?

Does he have any unusual experiences when going off to sleep?

Exactly what happens if the child will not go to bed or does not go to sleep readily? Who deals with the problem and how consistently?

Night-time

Does the child wake during the night? If so, when and how often? Does he get up in the night to go to the toilet or to have a drink? Is he able to return to sleep easily or does he need his parents or join them in their bed? If so, what precisely happens, who is involved and what is the result?

Is the child's sleep disturbed in other ways, e.g. restlessness, sleeptalking, sleepwalking, banging head or rocking, teeth grinding, nightmares or terrified episodes, jerking or convulsive movements or other episodes of disturbed behaviour? How often do these things occur, what time of night, how long do they last and does he seem awake at the time? What do the parents do?

Does the child snore or have any difficulty breathing when asleep?

Does he wet the bed?

Waking

What time does the child wake up? For how long has he slept?

Does he wake up spontaneously or have to be woken? Is it very difficult to wake him up? Does he look tired? Is he irritable and in a bad mood?

Does he have any unusual experiences and how does he feel between waking up and getting out of bed?

Table 5. (*cont.*)

Daytime

Is the child drowsy or does he sleep during the day? If he sleeps, can he resist doing so and does he fall asleep when engaged in activities?

What is the number, duration and timing of naps?

What is the total time spent asleep each 24 hours?

Do his muscles become weak when he laughs or is upset or surprised?

Does he find it difficult to concentrate?

Has his performance at school deteriorated?

Is he overactive, irritable or depressed?

Are there any other unusual episodes during the day?

Table 6. Basic principles of sleep hygiene

Sleeping environment should be conducive to sleep

Familiar setting

Comfortable bed

Correct temperature

Darkened, quiet room

Non-stimulating

No negative associations (e.g. punishment)

Encourage

Bedtime routines

Consistent bedtime and waking up times (weekdays, weekends, holidays within reason)

Going to bed only when tired

Thinking about problems and plans before going to bed

Falling asleep without parents (young children)

Regular daily exercise, exposure to sunlight, and general fitness

Avoid

Overexcitement near bedtime

Late evening exercise

Caffeine-containing drinks late in the day

Smoking and excessive alcohol (teenagers)

Large meals late at night

Excessive or late napping during the day

Too much time awake in bed (especially if distressed)

Date	Friday March 31st
Time woke/woken	7.00 am (woken by alarm)
Time got up	7.15 am
Any problems on waking? Please describe	Really sleepy-had to be dragged out of bed by Mum
Time and length of any daytime naps. What was your child doing just before he napped (e.g. at school, in the car, watching TV etc.)	2.10-2.20 pm. Fell asleep at school in maths lesson. Woken by teacher
Times during the day when your child seemed sleepy (although didn't nap). What was he doing at this time (e.g. at school, in the car, watching TV etc.)	He seemed a bit tired when he got home after school (3.45 pm). More lively after a little snack
Time to bed	8.15 pm
Time to sleep	9.30 pm
Any problems going to bed/getting off to sleep. Please describe including what you did, what your child did and how he eventually fell asleep.	He read until 8.30 pm. Light out. He came downstairs at 8.40 pm asking for a drink. Dad gave him a drink, took him back to bed & stayed with him until he fell asleep because he got upset when he tried to leave the room.
Time and length of any wakes during the night. Please describe why he woke (if known), what he did, what you did and how he eventually fell asleep.	2.20 am-heard him get up & go to the toilet. Seemed to go back to sleep within a few minutes-didn't call for Mum or Dad.
Times of breakfast (B), lunch (L), and dinner (D)	B 7.45 am L 12.30 pm D 5.45 pm
Anything else of importance (day or night)	He wasn't very well today. I think he's getting a cold.

Figure 2   Page from a sleep diary (with example).

situations (Johns, 1998), for use with children (Wiggs & Stores, 1995). Again, the value of such information is increased if it is collected from parents and children, and possibly other observers such as teachers.

Sleep diary (or sleep log)

Systematic recording each day over 2 weeks or more, using a standardized and simple format (see Figure 2), can provide valuable information about various aspects of sleep, avoiding the bias or distortion of retrospective generalizations especially by fraught parents.

- From a record of times of going to bed and getting to sleep, awake periods during the night, final awakening, getting up and (in young children) the details of daytime napping, the child's sleep–wake schedule and sleep rhythm can be assessed, together with estimates of total sleep time, sleep efficiency (proportion of time in bed the patient is actually asleep), and number of awakenings.
- The occurrence and nature of night-time episodes of disturbed behaviour can be determined.
- Daytime occurrences, including evidence of sleepiness, can be identified.
- Previously unrecognized sleep–wake patterns may become apparent, including shift of the sleep phase or relationships between sleep disturbance and stressful events or other factors.

Overall review

The following information is also needed in order to identify factors which might have contributed to the child's sleep problem:

- *medical and psychiatric history*, including past and current treatment details (in view of the wide range of illnesses or disorders and their treatment with which sleep disturbance is associated);
- *developmental history*, including perinatal and neonatal stages, predisposition to or evidence of developmental delay, educational history, adverse experiences at school or within the family:
- *social history*, including friendships, home and family circumstances, and recreational factors (drinking, smoking or drug use, especially in adolescents) which may affect sleep;
- *family history* (often positive in arousal disorders, enuresis and narcolepsy, for example);
- *system review of physical symptoms* to identify those associated with sleep disturbance, e.g. breathing difficulties or nocturia.

Physical and mental state examination

Particular attention should be paid to:

- evidence of any systemic illness which may disturb sleep, including neurological disorder or cardiorespiratory disease;
- obesity, facial or pharyngeal abnormalities, predisposing to upper airway obstruction in particular (chapter 5);
- overactivity, signs of depression or other psychiatric disorder;
- features of learning disability (including specific retardation syndromes) in view of its strong association with sleep disturbance.

Video recordings

Video recordings, preferably combined with audio recording, can be a valuable way of obtaining objective information about a child's sleep to supplement (or correct) descriptions provided in the clinic by parents. Especially when the night-time events are complex or dramatic (as in some of the parasomnias), parents' recall of them can easily be distorted or incomplete. It becomes difficult, therefore, to determine the precise sequence of events on which diagnosis should ideally be based. Sometimes, such recordings reveal a very different picture to that provided retrospectively in the clinic, especially concerning the parasomnias.

The recording can be performed in the child's home (using the family's own video system) or in nonspecialized settings such as a hospital ward, as distinct from a sleep laboratory. The child's sleep need not be disturbed if an infra-red camera or one sensitive to low light levels is used. A long-playing facility on the video recorder allows most if not all of the sleep period to be recorded. Parents often need advice on setting up the camera to obtain a useful view of the child. The recording should be as long as feasible, with the intention of recording through the episodes from their very beginning (the first changes can be the most instructive) rather than the camera being switched on when the parents hear a disturbance. Recording in these nonstandardized situations can be a hit-and-miss affair initially but, with perseverance, clinically useful information is usually possible.

Actigraphy

Monitoring of body movements during sleep is another relatively nonintrusive means of collecting objective information about sleep in nonlaboratory settings. A small wristwatch-type device is attached to the wrist or possibly a leg in younger children. A diary record is kept about the times the actometer is worn and when the child goes to bed and gets up. Scoring is done automatically to produce the type of analysis shown in Figure 3. Some information about healthy children is now available (Sadeh et al., 2000).

This kind of procedure has been used extensively and has been shown to agree closely with polysomnography for identifying basic patterns of sleep and wakefulness (American Sleep Disorders Association, 1995). Its relative simplicity makes it

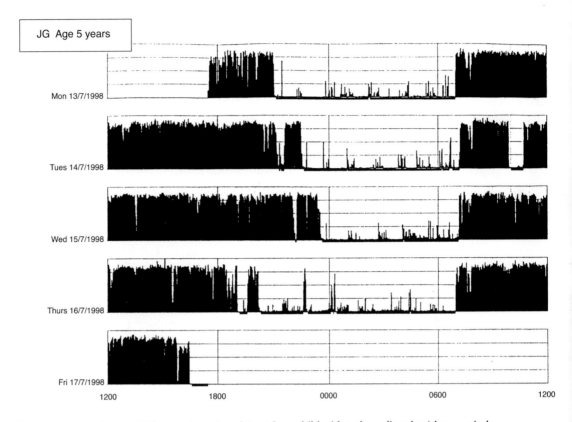

Figure 3   Continuous 95-hour actometry printout for a child with a sleep disorder (sleep periods underlined).

especially useful with children (Sadeh et al., 1991), where the details of sleep physiology are not needed as in disorders of the circadian sleep–wake cycle, although in children and adolescents five or more nights of recording are recommended to obtain reliable results (Acebo et al., 1999).

Polysomnography (PSG) (Broughton, 1999)

PSG provides information about the physiological changes that occur during sleep. *Basic PSG* entails recording of the EEG, EMG and the EOG. This allows the stages of sleep to be recognized according to the Rechtschaffen and Kales (1968) criteria to which reference was made earlier. A *hypnogram* is then compiled. Usually the recording is made overnight, but it may be extended to daytime if appropriate. Analysis of the results varies somewhat from one centre to another, but basic measures obtained from this information are as follows:

Sleep continuity
- Total time in bed (TIB)
- Time taken to go to sleep (sleep latency)
- Number of awakenings, possibly divided into brief awakenings (less than 2 minutes) and longer ones
- Time finally woke up
- Total time asleep
- Total time awake
- Sleep efficiency (total time in bed/total time asleep × 100)

NREM measures
- Actual and percentage time in stages 1–4
- Total slow wave sleep (SWS)

REM measures
- Time between first falling asleep and start of first REM period (REM latency)
- Actual and percentage time in REM sleep
- Total REM sleep

PSG extended to include additional physiological measures
- Respiratory variables (oronasal airflow, ribcage and abdominal movements, and blood gases) with audiovisual recording for *sleep-related breathing problems*. Detailed guidelines have been formulated for cardiopulmonary sleep studies in children (American Thoracic Society, 1996).
- Additional EEG channels (combined with video) if *nocturnal epilepsy* is suspected.
- Anterior tibialis EMG for the detection of *periodic limb movements in sleep* (*PLMS*).

Indications for PSG

PSG is necessary for diagnosis in only the minority of sleep disorders. The main indications for its use are as follows:
- The *investigation of excessive daytime sleepiness* (chapter 5), including the diagnosis of sleep apnoea, narcolepsy or PLMS. It is generally considered that (with the exception of young children) in such cases, the Multiple Sleep Latency Test (MSLT) (American Sleep Disorders Association, 1992) should be included. This quantifies daytime sleepiness by measuring the time the child takes to fall asleep during five opportunities (at 2-hourly intervals) to do so during the day. To avoid misleadingly unrepresentative results, the patient's sleep must have conformed to his usual pattern during at least the night before the test is performed,

and he must not be taking any medications acting on the central nervous system (CNS).

Some age-related normative data for laboratory PSG are available for children (Kahn et al., 1996). It appears that most children from the age of one upwards take at least 15 minutes to fall asleep in the sleep laboratory, and also during home polysomnography (Stores et al., 1998a), although there is much individual variation in both settings. The adult values are generally reached following puberty with some evidence that sleep latency (as well as total sleep time and daytime REM sleep latency values) vary according to the Tanner stage of sexual development (Carskadon & Dement, 1987). Even in the presence of sleep disorders usually characterized by excessive sleepiness, MSLT results can be normal in middle childhood because of the naturally enhanced daytime alertness at that age.

The Maintenance of Wakefulness Test (MWT), another objective measure of sleepiness sometimes used in adults but with less well-established normative data, requires the patient to remain awake as long as possible on repeated occasions.

The relative diagnostic value of the MSLT, MWT and the Epworth Sleepiness Scale has been debated with the view expressed that the ESS discriminates best between normal and pathological sleepiness (Johns, 2000).

- The *diagnosis of parasomnias* (chapter 6) in the following circumstances: where their nature is unclear from the clinical details; the episodes are unusual; there may be more than one type of parasomnia or another form of sleep disorder; the PSG findings contribute essentially to the diagnosis (notably REM sleep behaviour disorder); to determine the patient's state of wakefulness or sleep at the time of the episodes.
- As an *objective check* on the accuracy of the sleep complaint or response to treatment.
- To see if the patient is asleep during the clinical events. In the case of headbanging, for example, which can occur either before or during sleep, the findings will help to determine the choice of treatment. In other cases, sleep may be simulated for psychological reasons (Molaie & Deutsch, 1997).

Home polysomnography

Traditionally, PSG has entailed admission to a sleep laboratory where the recording environment and procedures are strictly controlled and standardized, including observations by a technician during the recording period. This 'laboratory PSG' has been viewed as the gold standard for physiological sleep studies. However, in many countries there are few such laboratories, and those that do exist are mainly designed for investigating adults. Sleep laboratories may make little if any concession to the special needs of children. Children's sleep laboratories should be particularly friendly and relaxed, and as far as possible free of frightening sights, sounds and smells. Staff should be experienced with children, and parents closely involved with facilities for mother staying overnight as appropriate.

In the absence of such facilities (although not solely for that reason), PSG at home (Stores, 1994) has much in its favour. Although used extensively in some centres, it is still generally underused. The procedure usually involves a small portable recording system (like a Walkman). This approach is not yet standardized to the extent of laboratory PSG, and for some sleep disorders it is best seen as a screening procedure. In its favour, especially for use with children, is that the patient can be investigated in real-life circumstances and without the recording procedure interfering with sleep and making the findings unrepresentative. If the recording is arranged with the full involvement and acceptance of the child, allowing sufficient time for him to become comfortable with the procedure by bedtime, the sleep disrupting first-night effects of the recording procedure (which are prominent in laboratory PSG) can be avoided or at least minimized (Palm et al., 1989; Kahn & Heckmatt, 1996). Systematic observations are important during the recording period. Normal values for children's home PSG are now available (Stores et al., 1998a).

Other investigations

Depending on the sleep disorder being considered, further laboratory investigations may be appropriate. These include:

- *haematological, biochemical and endocrine studies* especially in children who appear tired and lethargic;
- *urinalysis* in some cases of enuresis, or *toxicity screening* if substance abuse is suspected;
- *special EEG monitoring* as part of the investigations of possible epilepsy (Stores, 1985);
- *otolaryngological evaluation* in the case of upper-airway obstruction during sleep;
- *developmental assessment* if previously unidentified learning disability is suspected.

Treatment approaches for sleep disorders

The wide range of investigations that may be required illustrates the broad scope of children's sleep disorders medicine.

The same necessary breadth of vision is evident from the variety of possible treatments for sleep disorders which is underestimated in usual paediatric text-

Table 7. Examples of treatment approaches for sleep disorders

General principles

Explain the problem, reassure where appropriate and provide support

Encourage good sleep hygiene

Where possible treat any underlying cause of sleep disturbance

    Medical

    Psychiatric

Safety or protective measures (hazardous parasomnias)

Specific measures

Psychological (mainly for sleeplessness)

    Bedtime routine

    Positive associations with bedtime

    Promotion of self-soothing

    Setting limits

    Reinforcement of good behaviour

    Specific psychological treatments (e.g. gradual reduction of parental contact with the child at
        bedtime)

Chronobiological (circadian sleep–wake rhythm disorders)

    Sleep phase retiming

    Light therapy

Medication

    Hypnotics (selectively and short-term)

    Stimulants (excessive sleepiness)

    Melatonin (some circadian rhythm disorders)

Physical measures

    Continuous positive airway pressure (OSA)

Surgery

    Adenotonsillectomy (OSA)

book accounts. In clinical practice, pharmacological treatment is overemphasized, especially the use of hypnotic drugs (see chapter 4).

Table 7 provides some indication of the variety of available type of treatments, as well as general principles of management. The treatments are arranged roughly in order of the likely frequency of their use in a modern comprehensive sleep disorders service for children. An appropriate choice from this range requires an accurate diagnosis of the underlying sleep disorder. Claims for the effectiveness of these various measures are based on mainly clinical experience and reports. Few randomized controlled clinical trials have been published, as yet (see chapter 4).

The term '*sleep hygiene*' refers to 'conditions and practices that promote continuous and effective sleep' (American Sleep Disorders Association, 1997). Sleep hygiene principles are important at all ages, although the form that recommendations take obviously varies with the age of the individual and the circumstances. The recommendations listed in Table 6 cover general aspects, as well as others which are only relevant at particular ages from infancy to adolescence. A child's sleep problem may be wholly attributable to one or more aspects of poor sleep hygiene. In other cases, where there is a specific sleep disorder requiring its own treatment, good sleep hygiene can be an important additional part of overall management.

Melatonin requires a special mention because of its widespread popularity for many sleep disorders (Zhdanova, 2000). Clinical groups for which its effectiveness has been reported include multiply handicapped children, usually with severe visual impairment (Jan et al., 1994), and children with tuberous sclerosis (O'Callaghan et al., 1999), Rett syndrome (McArthur & Budden, 1998), Angelman syndrome (Zhdanova et al., 1999), and others with epileptic and nonepileptic myoclonus (Jan et al., 1999a). Ways in which children with neurodevelopmental disorders might be prone to melatonin abnormalities have been suggested by Zhdanova et al. (1999).

However, there is a need for further evaluation of the usefulness of melatonin in these and other childhood disorders by studies in which the nature of sleep disturbance is clearly specified, and the timing, dosage and other factors associated with success or failure are defined. In addition, long-term effects (both beneficial and troublesome, including possible effects on reproductive physiology) need to be assessed, as well as potential interactions with other forms of treatment. Without such studies it is difficult at present to evaluate adequately the place of melatonin in the treatment of sleep disorders. Certainly, it should not be viewed as the panacea that some reports imply.

Because of the aetiological differences discussed earlier (especially parental involvement), treatment often needs to be very different in children compared to adults. Appropriate psychological approaches usually entail alterations to parenting practices, designed to be acceptable and feasible in each individual family. Other forms of treatment, including chronobiological measures (adjustment of sleep schedules in circadian sleep–wake cycle disorders) also usually require considerable parental involvement. The same is true of general sleep hygiene principles. Explanation and (where appropriate) reassurance for the child and his parents are an essential part of any treatment, and are sometimes effective in their own right without the need for more specific measures.

4

Sleeplessness

General aspects

Definition of the problem

When parents say that they have a problem with their child's sleep it is essential to establish from the start the precise details of the problem as they see it. Doing so sometimes reveals that the child's sleep is actually within normal limits and that his parents (uncertain about children's sleep requirements including individual differences) are worried unnecessarily about possible harmful effects on their child of not getting enough sleep. In the circumstances, simple explanation and reassurance may be very therapeutic.

Assuming that the child's sleeplessness is 'real' rather than 'imaginary' in this sense, the following *types of sleeplessness* need to be distinguished from each other:
- *bedtime difficulties* (either *reluctance to go to bed* or *difficulty getting to sleep*);
- *waking up at night* and not being able to go to sleep again;
- *waking early in the morning*, not going back to sleep and causing a commotion.
The term 'sleeplessness' may also be used by parents to mean that their child's sleep is very restless or disturbed by frequent nightmares or other episodic events.

These problems may occur singly or combined. They need to be distinguished from each other because the factors causing or maintaining them can be different and may require different types of treatment.

Apart from its nature, sleeplessness can be defined in terms of its *severity*. Objectively, this includes the *frequency* with which the sleeplessness occurs, but this does not necessarily correspond to the seriousness of the problem as viewed by the parents. Different parents can tolerate the same degree of sleeplessness to very different extents, depending on their personality, emotional state and general circumstances. Clinically, their subjective view of the problem is what matters most, but some objective assessment also needs to be made if only to judge the degree of parental tolerance and to guide management.

A further dimension to the severity of sleeplessness (and, of course, other sleep problems) is its *duration*. This can be:

- *transient* (lasting several days), for example caused by a brief illness or the stress of an interview or examination;
- *short-term* (perhaps several weeks) such as that caused by illness or death within the family which, however, can cause much longer effects;
- *chronic* (months or years) caused by such problems as long-term physical illness or psychiatric disorder, or persistent circadian sleep–wake cycle disorders (see later).

Obviously, the help required depends very much on the underlying cause, and none may be needed for very brief, self-limiting conditions.

Prevalence

The general term 'sleeplessness' covers difficulty getting to sleep and/or staying asleep. 'Insomnia' tends to be used for those old enough to complain themselves about such problems. Sleeplessness is the main sleep problem at all ages from childhood to old age. In infants and toddlers alone, it is a source of concern to perhaps a quarter or more of families, with the possible consequences mentioned earlier for the child's psychological development, parental competence and well-being, and other aspects of family functioning (France & Hudson, 1993). In one form or another, sleeplessness continues to be common in older children and adolescents in the general population. Pollock (1994) described various forms of sleeplessness in about 25% of 5 year olds (although mostly of mild degree), Kahn et al. (1989a) reported mainly settling problems in 14% of 5–8 year olds and Morrison et al. (1992) described 15% of adolescents in the general population with difficulties getting to sleep or staying asleep. As emphasized earlier, sleeplessness is very frequently a significant additional difficulty for children who are chronically ill or disabled.

Severe settling and night-waking problems have been defined differently in different studies, giving rise to various prevalence rates all of which, however, are high (Blum, 1999). The ICSD criteria for severe 'sleep onset association disorder' are a prolonged sleep latency and, on at least 5 nights a week, waking either more than 3 times each night, or 2 or 3 times for over 10 minutes, or once for more than 15 minutes. Early waking is less consistently defined, and may well be judged differently from one family to another, but 5 a.m. or earlier has been used as a criterion (Simonds & Parraga, 1982). Reliable prevalence rates for this form of sleeplessness are not available.

Aetiology: general

Table 8 illustrates the wide range of factors that can underlie sleeping difficulties in children and adolescents. Clearly, many types of influence have to be considered in

Table 8. Factors to consider in sleepless children at different ages

Infancy
'Colic'
Cow's milk intolerance
Middle ear disease
Frequent nighttime feeds
Inappropriate sleep associations

Early childhood (1–3 years)
Inappropriate napping
Poor bedtime routine
Stressful or otherwise undesirable sleep onset associations
Poor limit setting
Too early bedtime

Middle childhood (4–12 years)
Difficulty getting to sleep
Persistence of earlier problems
Night-time fears
Overarousal
Worry and anxiety
Conditioned insomnia
'Owl' sleep–wake pattern
Idiopathic insomnia
Night waking
Parasomnias
Early morning waking
Advanced sleep phase syndrome
Reduced sleep requirements
Environmental disturbance
Conditioned early waking
'Lark' sleep–wake pattern
Constitutional 'short sleeper'

Adolescence
Worry and anxiety
Sleep-disrupting substances (recreational, illicit)
Circadian sleep–wake cycle disorders
Psychiatric disorder

explaining the individual case. Some are *physical* in nature, such as the medical conditions referred to particularly in infancy. These must not be overlooked by assuming that the explanation of the child's sleep problems lies in *parenting practices* which, however, are often important at any age but especially in early and middle childhood. In later childhood and adolescence, *personal, psychological and social factors* become more prominent.

Parenting and family issues

These feature prominently throughout childhood and into adolescence, in the origin, severity or the maintenance of sleep disturbance even where the basic cause is physical.

- Many settling and night-waking problems have their origins in parenting practices adjustment of which is the usual mainstay of successful treatment, as will be described shortly. Maternal factors associated with night waking in infants are thought to include general overconcern about the child's needs and health, possibly interacting with more demanding temperamental characteristics on the child's part (Blum, 1999), and sometimes originating in the mother's own parental attachment experiences as a child (Morrell, 1999).

  At a later stage, the way in which parents deal with their child's fears, worries and anxieties at bedtime will obviously influence the extent and duration of such concerns. Parents have a responsibility to encourage positive attitudes to sleeping rather than allow bedtime and sleep to become associated in the child's mind with distress or other negative feelings. Similarly, the adolescent's sleeping and waking patterns should not be a constant source of dispute and cause of alienation from his parents.

- Other aspects of family life may at least contribute to a child's failure to achieve or maintain satisfactory sleep habits, such as problems with other children in the family, marital discord, parental illness especially in mothers (Armstrong et al., 1998; Stoléru et al., 1997), bereavement or other loss including that of friends caused by a change of school or moving home, for example.

- In some families there is such disorganization in the way they function generally that, as part of this chaotic way of life, children develop a highly irregular sleep–wake pattern with no structure or consistency in either sleep or daytime behaviour. In these circumstances, there is likely to be a combination of bedtime difficulties, prolonged waking during the night, difficulty waking up, as well as underfunctioning and problem behaviour during the day which is partly the result of sleep disturbance.

Sleeping environment

In general, children seem to be more adaptable than adults to less than ideal sleeping conditions, although this is less so as they get older.

- Depending on family size and circumstances, a child may have to share a bedroom with other children who themselves have sleep problems, or the sleeping arrangements may be uncomfortable (too cold or too hot) or noisy because of the activities of other members of the family in close proximity.
- Various noisy activities on the part of parents can also disturb children's sleep, again depending on the layout of the house and the nature of the family's accommodation.
- The bedroom may be a very active place where the children play or talk with each other until late, or where a child with his own bedroom is in the habit of amusing himself with toys, television or computer.
- Noise from sources outside the home, such as nearby traffic, or morning light coming into the bedroom may be a problem.

Other aspects of sleep hygiene

Failure to observe sleep hygiene principles (especially in the setting of a generally disorganized way of family life) may result in complicated sleep disturbance including difficulty going to sleep, staying asleep and inappropriate sleep during the day, quite possibly with behavioural problems.

CASE: A 4-year-old boy was seen by his health visitor because of overactive behaviour during the day and settling and waking problems at night. Enquiries revealed that he regularly drank up to six cans of Coca Cola during the day and each evening he was put to bed with a large feeding bottle full of milky coffee. Precise calculation was not necessary to see that his daily caffeine intake was extremely high.

Most aspects of the family's life were described as ill-organized and unpredictable. Four of the 5 other children had behaviour problems, mother was said to be clinically depressed (mainly about financial problems) and father lived at home inconsistently.

Comment: Clearly, excessive caffeine intake is not confined to adolescents and adults. The effects of excessive caffeine seem to be the same in children as in adults including difficulty both in going off to sleep and staying asleep (Leibenluft, 1999). It might be thought that, with such a clear cause of his behaviour and sleeping difficulties, treatment would be straightforward. On the other hand, compliance problems were anticipated in such family circumstances in having the parents accept the advice that they were given. This proved to be so, and only a brief partial improvement was achieved. If, in contrast to this case, it is possible to introduce and maintain good sleep hygiene (and there is no other sleep disorder), a sustained improvement in the child's sleep can be expected.

Medical conditions

Although many forms of sleeplessness in children involve psychological factors and/or the effects of disturbed circadian rhythms, it is important to consider physical factors as a possible cause, whatever the age of the child. Sleeplessness caused by medical conditions is usually not confined to particular parts of the day, and is likely to be accompanied by failure to thrive or other evidence of physical disorder. Crying with failure to return to sleep despite attention from parents is also very suggestive that the child is physically distressed. Some conditions are seen in young children, others can occur at any age.

- *Cow's milk protein intolerance* should be considered as a cause of persistent sleeplessness in early infancy when no other cause is apparent, especially when there is a family history of atopy. Kahn et al. (1989b) have described an apparently close relationship in some infants between the ingestion of cow's milk and difficulty getting off to sleep, repeated wakening and crying, and overall reduction in the amount of sleep obtained by day and night. When awake, the child is likely to be sleepy and irritable. Other features of milk allergy (eczema, wheezing, gastrointestinal problems) may or may not be present. There may be immunoglobulin abnormalities (raised IgE and low IgA), raised eosinophil counts and skin reactivity, and the radioallergosorbent test (RAST) is likely to be positive for beta-lactoglobulin. There is usually a rapid response to the withdrawal of milk protein and an equally prompt relapse with its re-introduction. Treatment consists of replacing cow's milk in the night with tolerated protein. The condition usually remits spontaneously by the end of the first year.

- *Other food allergies* as a cause of behavioural disturbance (including sleep problems, but also skin rashes, breathing problems or gastrointestinal complaints) is a contentious topic but may be relevant in some children (Egger et al., 1992). Alternative possibilities should be considered, and this explanation only chosen if a close relationship can be demonstrated between the symptoms and ingestion of the foodstuff, including improvement when it is withheld.

- *Middle ear disease* is very common in childhood. Its acute form is readily recognized because of the pain and fever. In contrast, chronic middle ear disease is often insidious with few daytime symptoms but with sleep disturbance as possibly the only reported problem. Sleep may be affected because drainage of the fluid in the middle ear is further impaired when lying down, causing an increase in pressure and discomfort. The diagnosis may be suggested by a history of recurrent ear infections and evidence of middle ear disease on examination of the eardrums. Treatment consists of antibiotics or the insertion of drainage tubes, if necessary, following which sleep can be expected to improve.

- *Gastro-oesophageal reflux* is common in infancy with various degrees of severity. Nighttime symptoms can include frequent sudden awakenings, apnoeic episodes, delayed onset of sleep and more than usual sleepiness during the day (Ghaem et al., 1998).

- Other medical illnesses or disorders complicated by sleep disturbance were mentioned in chapter 2. These include *painful or uncomfortable conditions*, worsening of *asthma* during sleep, *nocturnal epilepsy,* various *other neurological disorders, upper airway obstruction, other systemic disease, medication effects* and *toxic states* resulting from medication overdosage or use of illegal substances. *Infantile colic* is usually listed as a cause of severe settling problems but, as will be discussed shortly, its standing as a medical entity is debated.

Genetic factors

Parkes (1999) and Zai et al., (2000) have reviewed the admittedly patchy evidence, so far, in favour of genetic factors in various human sleep disorders. These include some in which the main presentation is sleeplessness, such as insomnia of childhood or adolescent onset without any other obvious cause and some instances of delayed sleep phase syndrome or restless legs syndrome. Other sleep disorders for which some degree of genetic predisposition has been suggested are bruxism and (to a more significant extent) enuresis, arousal disorders and narcolepsy. In addition, a number of physical disorders of genetic origin give rise to sleep disorders, for example neuromuscular diseases causing obstructive sleep apnoea. In the case of sleeplessness, familial and other factors of a nongenetic nature are generally a much more likely explanation and should be sought, rather than assuming that the sleeping difficulty is somehow constitutional and difficult to change.

Treatment: general principles

There appears to be considerable room for improvement in the help provided to parents who seek advice for their child's sleep problems. For example, many parents expressed dissatisfaction with the help they received in Thunström's (1999) study of children in the general population. The problem is even greater for children with a learning disability (Wiggs & Stores, 1996).

The type of detailed history taking recommended earlier will usually suggest one or more reasons for a child's difficulty in sleeping. In theory, it should be possible to distinguish factors which:

- have been the fundamental *cause* of the difficulty;
- have consistently *precipitated* episodes of sleep disturbance (e.g. such distressing experiences as changing school, moving house, birth of a sibling, or illness or death within the family);
- have *maintained* the problem.

However, treatment appears to be most usefully based on factors maintaining the cause of the current sleep disturbance, rather than earlier causes or contributory factors.

From the diversity of factors listed in Table 8, it is clear that the treatment of sleeplessness varies considerably depending on its cause in the individual child. Based on careful description of the child's sleep disorder, a choice can be made from the various forms of treatment that were outlined in chapter 3. Often appropriate treatment will be psychological in nature, rarely pharmacological. General principles of sleep hygiene are often advisable and, of course, attention to any underlying physical or psychological disorder in the child or his parents.

Medication

The use of medication requires further comment in view of the frequency with which it is still prescribed, especially for young children whose parents complain about their sleep. Its use is generally the result of not considering the underlying cause of the problem and desperation on the part of parents and physicians unfamiliar with effective behavioural alternatives.

Antihistamines, chloral-containing preparations and benzodiazepines are used, despite the lack of sound evidence that they are effective. Review of randomized controlled trials of interventions for settling and night-waking problems indicates that medication (often in the form of trimeprazine) appears to be effective in the short-term for night waking in children under 6 years, but its long-term efficacy is highly questionable (Ramchandani et al., 2000). Apart from other considerations, medication is not popular with parents and is likely to interfere with the child learning to fall asleep unaided.

On this basis, the use of medication might be justified only occasionally as a short-term measure to ensure a few nights sleep before psychological measures are started. A sufficiently large dose of chloral hydrate or trimeprazine should be used to ensure this respite; a tentative dose is likely to induce a confusional state at bedtime and make the child more distressed. Another possible use of short-term sedation is in combination with a psychological approach to treatment for settling and night-waking problems in young children (described later) but this is not a well-validated practice.

It should not be assumed that medication will necessarily be needed in children with neurodevelopmental disorders thought to be the basic cause of sleeping difficulties. Behavioural treatments can be quickly effective in such children as discussed later in this chapter.

Developmental approach

Although in the following account (for ease of reference) different forms of sleeplessness, and the underlying causes and contributory factors, are arranged in developmental sequence, these age distinctions should not be interpreted too strictly as there is often overlap from one stage of development to another. At any age, sleep may be disturbed in more than one way.

Infancy

Excessive crying in infants and infantile colic

This commonly worries parents of young infants, many of whom are taken to their health visitor or family doctor for the problem. It is often associated with sleeping problems. In particular, '*infantile colic*', usually starting at 2–3 weeks of age, is seen as a common cause of difficulty settling otherwise healthy babies in the evening (Weissbluth, 1995b). The traditional view has been that this condition is fundamentally an intestinal disorder causing paroxysms of pain and intense inconsolable crying (mainly between 5 p.m. and midnight) with stiffening, drawing up of the legs and writhing as if in pain. Its reported response to antispasmodic drugs has reinforced this view, although its physical basis has not been confirmed by investigation. Typically, the intense crying resolves spontaneously in about 3–4 months. However, it is thought that sleep problems may then continue because the child has come to expect considerable attention from his parents in the evening and depends on their presence to get to sleep.

In fact, the nature and significance of infantile colic is disputed, and there is some doubt that it is an intestinal problem distinct from other patterns of crying in infants (St James-Roberts et al., 1996). Gormally & Barr (1997) consider that at most 5–10% of infants whose crying comes to medical attention have some form of organic cause characterized by convincing features of physical abnormality. Neither the usual 'colicky' child's behaviour when crying, nor the timing of the crying are thought to be necessarily very different from other children who cry a great deal, and there is some evidence that the crying may be at least partly temperamental in origin (Canivet et al., 2000). Helping parents to cope with the crying has been advocated for most cases, rather than trying to treat it specifically with antispasmodic drugs (St James-Roberts, 1992).

Nighttime feeds

If a baby wakes frequently at night and will only return to sleep by being fed (perhaps with only a few sucks), it is likely that he has become conditioned to waking repeatedly because he is hungry and needs to be fed in order to get back to sleep. A healthy, full-term baby should be capable of confining feeding to daytime by 6 months of age if not earlier, but establishing this pattern will be hindered by frequent night-time feeding on demand, especially if large amounts of fluid are consumed by the baby making him uncomfortable from very wet nappies. Being fed at each awakening also makes attention from his mother a condition for the infant being able to get back to sleep.

Some mothers may value the child's need for them during the night. However, if help is requested, treatment consists of gradually reducing the frequency of night-time feeds, the amount of fluid provided at each feed and time spent feeding. If necessary, mothers may be convinced that the baby is not really hungry by showing that a feed of diluted milk (or even water) is sufficient to settle him. In children of an appropriate age, it should be possible to eliminate the nighttime feeds and sleep disturbance within about 1–2 weeks.

Giving a feed when the infant wakes up early in the morning should be avoided, as this will reinforce early waking because of feelings of hunger at that time. Again, gradually delaying the time of that first feed of the day should help to delay the time the child wakes up. Practical advice for parents on these aspects of infant feeding is provided by Ferber (1986).

Parents sometimes attribute sleep problems from about 6 months onwards to *teething*, but the connection has been difficult to confirm (Macknin et al., 2000). It is an unlikely explanation for such problems lasting weeks or longer.

Early childhood (1–3 years)

Napping

Difficulties at bedtime may be the result of an inappropriate pattern of napping during the day compared with the usual pattern which varies with age, as described previously. A child will not be ready to settle to sleep at the time preferred by his parents if the last nap is close to bedtime, or if it is earlier in the afternoon but long. Alternatively, the problem may be that too many naps are being taken or that there is a disproportionate amount of the total 24 hours of sleep being taken during the day. The opposite of this, but with similar results, occurs when the child does not sleep enough in the daytime with the result that he is 'overtired', irritable and too active at bedtime.

Inappropriately timed daytime naps may cause not only difficulty getting to sleep, but early waking if the first nap of the day is unusually early in the morning. In fact, this nap may represent the last sleep cycle which has become detached from the rest of the overnight sleep period. Progressively delaying the time of the first nap, and (by degrees) not attending to the child when he wakes up until a later time, should help him fall asleep again by himself after a short period.

Changes in the timing of napping need to be made gradually by steps of about 10–15 minutes. Ways of changing the pattern of napping are also well described for parents by Ferber (1986).

'Behavioural' settling and waking problems: general

The most common sleep problem (of which many parents are only too well aware) is *difficulty getting their child to settle to sleep* at bedtime, often accompanied by demands for their attention when the child *wakes at night*. As mentioned earlier, this happens frequently in 20% or more of children between the ages of about 1 and 3 years. The effects on the child, his parents and other children in the family can be serious because of sleep loss and strained relationships between parent and child.

Such problems should not be viewed as an inevitable part of having young children; they can be helped considerably. Unfortunately, the correct form of treatment and advice is often not provided. It is important to deal with such problems at an early stage (or ideally to prevent them occurring in the first place) not only because of the immediate difficulties for the child and the family to which they give rise, but also because of the risk that they may lay the foundations for later sleep disturbance and other behavioural problems. Nevertheless, even when the sleep problem is long-standing, psychological treatments can be effective.

Recommendations for bedtime

There are a number of ways in which parents might be able to prevent or minimize these settling and night-waking problems. The principles involved also form the basis of the behavioural treatment programmes that are likely to be useful where such difficulties have become established.

- A consistent *bedtime routine* and '*wind down*' *period* is highly desirable consisting of a sequence of evening events (i.e. feeding, bathing, stories and close contact with parents) with a definite end point at which the child should be relaxed enough to go to sleep, allowing parents time to themselves for the rest of the evening.
- This routine, and the child's sleeping environment (including the bedroom, cot or bed, favourite toys or other comforting objects), should establish '*sleep onset associations*' that are conducive to sleep. Being in bed should not be associated in the child's mind with play or other stimulating activities, and certainly not with punishment or other upsetting experiences.

  From early infancy the positive associations of actually going to sleep, however, should preferably not include being downstairs or held, rocked, nursed or being in the parents' bed, as this close contact (usually with mother) becomes a necessary condition for getting back to sleep when the child wakes during the night. Infants are more likely to have difficulty settling back to sleep after waking up at night if their parents are present when they fall asleep at bedtime (Adair et al., 1991). Similarly, the use of a dummy (or 'pacifier') to help an infant to settle can be unhelpful when the child loses contact with it during the night. For this and other reasons, including possible interference with breast feeding, the wisdom of using a dummy is still much debated (Winberg, 1999).

  Waking at night is normal at all ages. Infants (even those who are said to sleep well) wake several times throughout the night from both REM and NREM sleep.

In the next few years, waking occurs mainly in the middle period of overnight sleep when sleep is not at its deepest levels. Many infants cry when they awake (so-called '*signallers*') but from about 6 to 12 months of age most are capable of returning to sleep without needing their parents' attention ('*self-soothers*').

A problem arises if the child cannot go to sleep at bedtime or (more especially) if he cannot get back to sleep after waking in the night without the comforting presence of a parent or any other associations that the child cannot readily achieve without the parent's help (e.g. certain play activities). The child's need for his parents during the night can be avoided if the child falls asleep at bedtime in the same circumstances (in particular without his parents' presence) as he will experience when he wakes during the night.

CASE: A 4-year-old boy was very distressed at bedtime unless one of his parents was in the room with him until he fell asleep. When he woke at night, he again needed his parents to pacify him in order to get back to sleep. The settling difficulty was not too disruptive to the family since he fell asleep within a few minutes with a parent sitting beside his bed, but the night waking had become a main concern since the arrival of a new baby.

As father frequently worked away from home, he was not always available to help with the children either at bedtime or when they woke in the night. Mother was not hopeful about being able herself to carry through any behavioural programme, especially in the middle of the night when she felt very weary. In these circumstances, it was suggested that mother (and also father when he was available) should deal first with the boy's settling problems and teach him to fall asleep at bedtime and to continue resettling him during the night, as before, by going into his bedroom when he called out for them.

The parents chose to use the checking method (see later) and after 6 days the boy was settling to sleep unaided. As he learnt to settle himself to sleep, the frequency of his night waking began to lessen and within 2 weeks had resolved without any further type of treatment.

Comment: Where children have both settling and night-waking problems it is often possible to deal with both problems simply by addressing the settling difficulties. If the child can be taught how to fall asleep without his parents being present, this learned ability may well be transferred to later in the night when the child wakes up. This approach may be particularly appropriate for parents who have additional stresses and may not feel able to cope with any procedure which initially means further loss of sleep.

- *Bedtime struggles* because of the child's reluctance to go to bed (as distinct from inability to fall asleep) are commonplace, especially when the child moves from cot to bed and is no longer easily constrained. Many parents are familiar with bedtime delaying tactics in which their child asks for drinks, more stories or cuddles, expresses fear at the prospect of bed, or steadfastly refuses to go to bed, perhaps with tantrums or other forms of difficult behaviour. Once asleep, the child may then sleep soundly.

Often the problem is maintained or made worse by parents' inability or unwillingness to establish and consistently enforce rules for going to bed and settling to sleep ('*setting limits*'). A clue to the nature of the problem can be the child's willingness to settle with one parent rather than the other, or with the babysitter or someone else who does set limits to the child's behaviour. The unhelpful effects of the parents' inability to set limits are compounded if they lose their temper, threaten or punish the child who then comes to associate bedtime with upset and fear. Parents who have marital or other psychological difficulties are more likely to behave inappropriately if their child resists going to bed.

The basic aim of preventing or discouraging difficult behaviour at bedtime is to introduce a consistent limit setting procedure. Reinforcement of the problem behaviour by giving in to the child's demands must be avoided. A bedtime routine and wind down period are important, with established rules which the child understands. Removing uncertainty from the situation can itself be reassuring to the child enabling him to relax instead of struggle. Appropriate reward systems, consistently applied for good behaviour, also have their place once the child is old enough to understand them.

• Setting limits is only appropriate if the child is physiologically capable of going to sleep at the required time. Many children and adults have a period later in the day when their tendency towards sleep is at its lowest, i.e. the '*forbidden zone*' (Lavie, 1986) when the child gets its '*second wind*'. This is followed by a period of reducing alertness leading to the onset of sleep. If a child is habitually put to bed while still wide awake (i.e. while still in the forbidden zone), he will resist, perhaps vigorously. A clue to this state of affairs is that he will eventually fall asleep at the same time each night, irrespective of the time at which attempts to put him to bed are started.

It is easy to see how the child's physiological inability to go to sleep can be misinterpreted as naughtiness. The distinction can be difficult to make, but the possibility that the child's bedtime is too early should be considered and the sequence of events leading up to bedtime arranged so that the child goes to bed when '*sleepy tired*'. This allows going to bed to become associated with falling asleep quickly rather than with lying awake, struggles with parents or other negative experiences. If getting up for nursery or school is then particularly difficult, bedtime can be very gradually brought forward to the point where the child wakes up spontaneously or can easily be woken at the right time.

The problem of too early a bedtime is greater in children who are constitutionally *owls* in the timing of their sleep phase, with their highest level of alertness later in the evening compared with other children. There may be limited prospects of changing this pattern which, therefore, has to be accommodated by parents. However, in the majority of children it is possible to alter the timing of their sleep to some extent.

Treatment possibilities and parental involvement

If the happy state of affairs in which the child readily settles to sleep at the right time for his parents and does not disturb them during the night has not been achieved, and he is consistently difficult to settle or is distressed when he wakes up during the night, treatment is required. As mentioned already, medication is very rarely the solution.

There are various forms of psychological treatment which have been shown to be effective. Some can be called '*behavioural*' in applying basic learning theory principles to change the child's behaviour. '*Cognitive–behavioural*' methods implies accompanying changes in the child's thoughts, attitudes or beliefs when his level of development makes this possible. Even purely behavioural treatments usually involve some degree of cognitive change on the parents' part.

The choice of treatment depends principally on the individual family for which treatment needs to be designed in the light of the particular problem, and also what the parents are capable of or willing to do. The practical details of their use have been provided by Edwards & Christopherson (1994) and France et al. (1996). Owens et al. (1999a) and Ramchandani et al. (2000) have examined the general evidence for the effectiveness of such measures. Likewise, Wiggs & France (2000) have reviewed behavioural treatments in children and adolescents with physical illness, psychological problems and learning disability, while Lancioni et al. (1999) have assessed the evidence for their efficacy more specifically in people with a learning disability or multiple disabilities. Fuller accounts are contained in books for parents by Douglas & Richman (1984), Ferber (1986) and Quine (1997).

For a psychological approach to have a chance to work, it is necessary for parents to see their child's sleep disturbance as a problem, to be given sufficient confidence that treatment can be effective, and to be able to commit themselves to the effort and persistence that is required. Sometimes parents are unsure about undertaking such treatment because they feel that competent parents should be able to cope without any special help, or they may be confused by conflicting advice from various sources. They may well feel guilty about not readily agreeing to their child's need for them at night, especially if his demands intensify in the early phase of treatment. In all these circumstances, parents need to be convinced of the benefits to the child and themselves of improving his sleep habit.

There are other possible reasons why parents are unwilling to be involved in a treatment programme, or why they fail to see it through. Each will require attention before treatment can proceed or be expected to be effective.

- Parents may be disenchanted by past failed attempts at treatment which, on enquiry, turn out to have been inappropriately chosen and implemented. Hopefully, explanation will restore their confidence enough for them to try again.

CASE: The parents of an 11-year-old girl with microcephaly and severe learning disability reported that she had never slept well and even as a baby had woken nearly every hour for long periods. Since starting to walk, she had often left her room after waking up and wandered about the house sometimes injuring herself. When she was 3 her parents tried using hypnotic medication but did not persist because it made her drowsy during the day. As attempts to return her to her room when she woke in the night were unsuccessful, they resorted to taking her into their bed.

At the time of referral to the sleep disorders clinic, the child still woke every night between 2 and 3 a.m. and came into her parents' bed where she slept until morning. They were sceptical about any psychological approach because they had tried such treatments previously without success and thought this meant that their child's sleep pattern was an untreatable part of her general condition. However, being desperate, they agreed to try again by returning the child to her own bed when she came into their room at night. The therapist warned them to expect an initial worsening of the problem when treatment began.

On the first night she was taken back to her bed and told to go to sleep there, which she did quickly and without upset. She came out of her room again later that night but, again, was readily settled back in her own bed. The night after was the same, but on the third night she stayed in her room and continued to do so from then on. Occasionally she would call out if she woke up, but the parents were able to simply call back reassuringly which was sufficient for her to go back to sleep again. Soon she stopped calling out at night altogether.

Comment: Response to treatment in this case was particularly rapid and effective. The case illustrates that, as for healthy children, children with learning disabilities need to be told and shown how they are expected to sleep. Once shown a new set of behaviours, the child readily accepted the situation. The case also illustrates that psychological interventions which have been unsuccessful at one stage can be helpful at a later date. In fact, inquiry revealed that the earlier advice about psychological treatments had not really been followed for lack of professional support and the parents' belief that their daughter's difficult behaviour was an inevitable part of her neurological disability.

- Parents may be emotionally incapable of meeting the demands of the treatment programme because they are overwhelmed by other problems.
- The possibility was mentioned earlier that, in fact, parents may not want the situation to change in spite of apparent difficulties caused by the child's sleep disturbance. A mother may need to maintain her child's dependence on her in the absence of other ways of meeting her own emotional needs. A child's presence in his parents' bed may be welcomed by one of the partners because it limits intimate contact with the other.
- Parents may be understandably concerned about their child coming to harm if

he has an illness or disorder which might need attention at night, such as
epilepsy or asthma. For such children in particular, treatments that involve
ignoring the child's cries at night are inappropriate.

- As illustrated earlier, some families have such a generally disorganized way of life
  that it is beyond them to undertake a systematic programme of treatment.
  Failure to comply with requests to complete a sleep diary may well suggest that
  this is so. There may be little that can be done in such circumstances.

Types of psychological approach

These can be grouped as:
- ways of 'setting the scene' for sleep;
- promotion of self soothing by the child;
- scheduled awakenings;
- rewarding good behaviour.

Setting the scene

Several ways of doing this were mentioned as recommendations for bedtime,
especially having a consistent wind-down bedtime routine, avoiding too early a
bedtime and instead putting the child to bed when ready to sleep, and building up
relaxing and pleasurable associations with going to bed. These measures (sometimes referred to as '*stimulus control*') are valuable in their own right but can also
be important as a part of more specific psychological treatment programmes. The
same is true of some of the sleep hygiene principles described in chapter 3.

Ways of promoting self-soothing

Specific psychological treatments are required if the child cannot settle to sleep
alone, or is unable to return to sleep after waking in the night without attention
from his parents.

A basic feature of treatments which involve ignoring the child is that the sleep
disturbance must not be reinforced by the active presence of the parents. Interaction between parent and child, therefore, is reduced to a minimum. The
routines suggested should be followed consistently whenever the child should be
falling asleep, i.e. at bedtime, following awakening during the night and also when
daytime naps are due. However, it is usually advisable to start with one of these
situations and to deal with the other later. For example, if a child has both settling
and night-waking problems, parents are advised to concentrate on his bedtime
behaviour and then to move on to the night waking as their confidence grows.
Each form of treatment has its strengths and weaknesses.

(1) *Systematic ignoring* (*or* '*extinction*') (France & Hudson, 1990). Typically, to
settle the child, a short bedtime routine is followed. The child is put in his cot or

bed, parents say 'good night' and leave the room. The parents do not go back to the child (unless they fear he is ill or in danger) until the morning. In the case of night waking, the parents go to the child when they first hear him crying, check that he is not ill, change his nappy in the cot if necessary, but do not pick up, soothe, interact or feed the child in any way. They then leave the room and do not return during the crying episode. Further episodes of crying are dealt with in the same way.

This method is said to be rapidly effective over a matter of only a few days, but many parents are too distressed or feel too guilty to persist with it. Indeed, it is ill-advised if a child has a medical condition that might worsen at night. It is also not practical if there are other members of the family (and even neighbours) who are likely to be disturbed because the child's sleep problem and crying usually get worse before they improve.

(2) *Variations on complete ignoring*, which are generally more acceptable, involve various ways in which parents gradually reduce their reinforcing contact with the child when he cries (*'fading'*). As there is some empirical support for the use of all these measures, the choice depends largely on parents' preference in the light of what they can best manage to achieve. It may be necessary to try different approaches in turn to establish which is the most acceptable, but each should be attempted with as much determination as possible, rather than abandoning the procedure half tried.

- *Gradual reduction of proximity to the child* (Minde et al., 1994). The parent gradually reduces the physical proximity to the child over subsequent nights and weeks, for example moving from lying down with the child, to sitting on his bed, next sitting on a chair at the side of the bed, and then moving the chair gradually further away from the child. All forms of interaction with the child should be avoided.
- *Gradual reduction of time spent with the child* (Lawton et al., 1991). Over about a 1-month period, the parent gradually increases the time before responding to the child, or reduces the time spent with him each time he cries. These approaches are said to be very effective. They are also acceptable to parents who are sufficiently committed and well organized to undertake this extended programme.
- *Gradual reduction of reinforcement in other ways* (Ferber, 1986), for example, contact with the parent is made gradually less rewarding by substituting water for milk when the infant demands a bottle.
- *Checking* (Pritchard & Appleton, 1988). When the child cries, the parent checks him about every 10 minutes to briefly reassure him but without doing anything more. The time interval can be adjusted according to parents' preference. Some parents choose to start with very brief intervals between checks (e.g. one minute)

and to gradually increase the time by 1–2 minutes. This is also said to be rapidly effective although, initially, crying may become more intense each time the parent makes contact.

- *Ignoring with parents remaining in the room* (Sadeh, 1994). When the child cries the parent stays in his room (with low illumination or some other way, such as the occasional cough, of letting him know that the parent is present) and remains there, ignoring the crying, until the child is asleep. The parent returns as soon as the child wakes up and cries, and follows the same procedure. This method is said to have the advantage that it decreases the child's crying and the parents' anxiety, and is reported to be effective within perhaps a week. However, it is obviously inconvenient and allows the child to become self-soothing to only a limited extent.
- Some success has been reported with a combination of short-term (10 days) trimeprazine and the ignoring procedure (France et al., 1991). Its advantages are said to be a reduction of the child's distress and parental anxiety, again with a fairly rapid response. However, many parents object to the use of medication.

Scheduled awakening (Rickert & Johnson, 1998)

This rather surprising procedure has been used for night waking without settling problems. It refers to systematically waking the child (usually an infant) before the time he usually wakes (as determined by prior observations) in order to feed or soothe him. The rationale is that waking the child in this way reduces the likelihood of spontaneous wakings. The frequency of the awakenings is gradually reduced until they are discontinued completely. The appeal of this procedure is limited for parents who see the awakenings as intrusive to the child and trouble-some for themselves.

Rewarding good behaviour

For children old enough to understand them, *reward systems*, such as a star chart (used consistently and immediately after the behaviour being encouraged), can be effective in addition to one or other of these specific psychological treatments. Sometimes it is an effective measure by itself.

It may be appropriate to combine different elements to tailor a treatment programme for the individual child.

CASE: An 18-month-old girl was referred by her family doctor because her disturbed sleep was causing much upset in the family. The child's early development had been otherwise normal, although she was a hungry baby and was fed 2-hourly at night for the first few months. Settling to sleep was not a problem but by 6 months of age she was waking and screaming for attention about 2 a.m. every night. Sedation had been prescribed but had no effect.

Similarly, no improvement was achieved by setting a bedtime routine, providing a comforting piece of material from her mother's clothes and by mother sleeping on the child's bedroom floor. She could only tolerate ignoring her child's cries for one night.

On the basis of information contained in a 2-week sleep diary, the night-time feeds given to help the child settle back to sleep were gradually discontinued and the child was encouraged to settle herself back to sleep by stepwise extending the time between each waking and mother attending to her daughter. Mother was also encouraged to have minimum contact when the child woke, simply reminding her daughter that it was time to sleep before leaving the room. Weekly telephone contact was maintained with mother to help ensure that these measures were employed consistently. Within 4–5 weeks, the waking problem had been resolved with no recurrence over the following 3 years.

Comment: Depending on the parents' capabilities and circumstances, a gradual approach to treatment may be much more preferable and feasible despite taking longer to have an effect.

Parental confidence and motivation

As emphasized already, choice of psychological approaches depends on what is acceptable and possible for a given family. Defining the appropriate treatment programme requires close co-operation between the health visitor, psychologist or other professional adviser and the parents. *Support and encouragement* is also needed by parents to see the programme through. This is especially the case if progress seems slow or there are setbacks such as temporary worsening of the problem (which not infrequently occurs at the start of treatment or even after an initial period of improvement), or if the child is ill for a time or relapses for some other reason. Parents may also need professional support in the face of criticism from other people, including grandparents, who may suggest various homespun remedies.

Ideally, improvement in the child's sleep will be maintained in the long-term. Therefore, *follow up* is an essential part of the treatment process with parents able to make contact in the meantime, as necessary. However, should relapse occur, the demonstration to parents that the problem can be treated, and that they can again be in control of the situation, should give them the confidence to start the treatment programme again.

The available evidence suggests that, carefully chosen and implemented consistently and with determination, psychological treatment for settling and waking problems can be very effective in a short period of time, even in children with severe and long-standing problems and with serious neurodevelopmental disorders (Piazza et al., 1997; Wiggs & Stores, 1998).

CASE: A 6-year-old girl with severe developmental delay of unknown cause had challenging daytime behaviour, taking the form of prolonged screaming, temper tantrums, aggression and food refusal. Her parents found coping with this behaviour increasingly difficult, especially since she also had severe sleep problems which disrupted their own sleep constantly. The child's health was generally good apart from infrequent generalized tonic–clonic seizures for which she was taking medication.

The child was said to have never slept well since birth. The current problems, which had been present since age 2, were refusal to go to bed and waking in the night. She insisted on remaining downstairs with her parents who held her until she fell asleep (very late) and then carried her up to bed. She woke every night in the early hours of the morning and came into her parents' bed for the remainder of the night but taking 1–2 hours to go back to sleep again.

A number of different sedative medications had been tried without success. A psychological programme which involved ignoring her had been abandoned because of the crying and loud screaming which the parents found very distressing. It was also unacceptable because the other children were woken by her screams.

A more graded psychological approach was devised aimed at teaching the child to fall asleep alone at an appropriate time, and to know that her bedroom was the room in which she should sleep. A downstairs bedtime routine was devised leading to the time she usually fell asleep. After a few days this was easily transferred upstairs to her bedroom. The routine was then gradually brought forward by 10 minutes or so every other night until she was falling asleep at an appropriate time. Over successive nights, mother then gradually distanced herself during settling by standing further and further away from the bed, until eventually she was out of the room.

Five weeks after starting this programme, the child was happily going upstairs at bedtime and could be quickly settled by her mother who was then able to leave the room. Without any direct intervention, her night waking also improved. Because she had learned to settle herself to sleep at bedtime, the child resettled herself if she woke in the night. About once a week she woke up and called to her mother or went into her room, but readily went back to her own bed when her mother simply asked her to do so.

Mother reported an improvement in the child's daytime behaviour which she attributed to sleeping better and having less fraught nights. The child was less aggressive and irritable, and cried and screamed much less during the day. Mother also said that she herself felt much better in general because she was sleeping well at night and had her evenings free to spend with her husband.

Comment: This case illustrates that severe learning disability, epilepsy and seriously disturbed behaviour are not necessarily a barrier to the successful use of psychological treatment for a child's sleep disorder. It also demonstrates that significant improvement in general behaviour can be associated with better sleep to the benefit of the family as a whole.

Middle childhood (4–12 years)

In general, children at this stage of development have fewer problems going to sleep or staying asleep compared with younger children or adolescents. Where there is a problem, it mainly takes the form of difficulty settling to sleep. Less often, the problem is waking up too early, at least from the point of view of other members of the family.

Apart from inappropriate napping, some of the causes of sleeplessness in toddlers and their treatment still apply in older children. In particular, setting limits at bedtime (discussed earlier) may still be necessary to deal with repeated requests and excuses for not going to bed. However, other factors become more relevant with increasing age.

Difficulty getting to sleep

- If a child is *overaroused* at bedtime it may be difficult for him to get to sleep or stay asleep. Boisterous activities, exciting or frightening stories or television programmes before going to bed should be discouraged. This problem is often worse where children share a bedroom. It has been reported that the presence of a television set in the child's bedroom is an important contributory factor in children's sleep problems, including resistance to go to sleep and delay in getting to sleep (Owens et al., 1999b).
- *Night-time fears* (King et al., 1997) are common from very early childhood onwards and are quite likely combined with the anxiety that children might feel at being separated from their parents at night. Children may have an aversion to being in their bedroom at night and insist on the room being lit or sleeping with their parents.

As development progresses, the content of the fears changes with age. Initially, the fears may involve aspects of the immediate environment (shadows, noises etc.), then later imaginary objects (ghosts, monsters) or the dark. These give way to more specific worries (Muris et al., 2000) which may involve the child's own health, or his parents coming to harm in the night for example. Such fears and worries are usually transient and require only reassurance and comfort until they fade, but in some children they are so intense and persistent that they reach phobic proportions and need special attention.

The cause of the fear should be explored. Fears may be triggered by a traumatic event, such as loss of a relative or friend. It may be one aspect of an anxiety state, including post-traumatic stress disorder, in which case the child might also suffer from parasomnias such as nightmares. The content of the fear or nightmare might be revealing. If fears and nightmares are frequent, particularly disturbing or if the child cannot be reassured, a serious underlying cause should be considered such as family disruption or other psychological stress. Other sleep disturbances (e.g. alarming hypnagogic hallucinations) or the prospect of disturbing experiences caused by physical illness (such as nocturnal asthma attacks) might instill fear in the child at bedtime.

A child's reluctance to go to bed because he is genuinely afraid must be distinguished from pretending to be afraid as a delaying tactic.

Treatment depends on the intensity of the fear and whether it is part of a more general condition needing psychiatric treatment in its own right. In milder cases (at this age and earlier) subdued lighting in the bedroom or a comforting toy might help. Severe upset requires more specific measures. If the fear is relatively isolated, psychological approaches can be effective. These include encouraging self-control by means of relaxation techniques, combating the fear by substituting pleasant images, displacing fear by other emotions, or boosting self-confidence. These measures, and also systematic desensitization (gradual exposure to the frightening situation) and reward systems, have all been reported to have lasting beneficial effects (Owens et al., 1999a). Other measures for older children include training in ways of counteracting irrational beliefs. The fearful child will be helped by positive associations with bedtime and not going to bed so early that he lies awake in a fearful state.

- Difficulty getting to sleep (and disturbed sleep) may be caused by *stress, worry or upset* about family issues (illness, separation from parents, arrival of a new baby, other sibling rivalry, death of a pet, moving house, marital problems) or school problems (poor progress, bullying, starting or changing school). Some children have to complete a ritualistic sequence of actions before they can relax enough to go to sleep. The need to do this is greater, more prolonged and accompanied by other abnormal behaviours in obsessive–compulsive states. Reactions to severe stress are likely to involve more than sleep disturbance. Characteristically the child will have other complaints, including other signs of anxiety and quite possibly physical symptoms such as headaches or other physical complaints.

  Sympathetic discussion of the child's worries, attention to the source of concern and ways of helping the child to relax at night (e.g. by making before bedtime a 'worry list' of daytime issues which might cause concern when lying in bed) are generally thought to help. More specific psychiatric measures will be needed if the child has an anxiety or depressive disorder, other psychiatric illness, or if there is evidence of serious problems within the family.

- The original source of anxiety may no longer exist, but the difficulty in falling asleep may persist because the child or adolescent has developed the habit of lying awake in bed in an agitated state ('*conditioned* or *learned insomnia*').

- The '*owlish*' *type sleep–wake pattern* in which the child is particularly alert late into the evening, was mentioned earlier.

- '*Idiopathic insomnia*' (or *childhood onset insomnia*) refers to another constitutional condition in which there is a lifelong difficulty sleeping, including getting off to sleep, which is not attributable to environmental, emotional or medical factors and therefore assumed to be constitutional in origin. The diagnosis is usually made retrospectively in adult life. It is important not to assume a constitutional cause of any sleeping difficulty but to enquire about other more likely explanations.

Waking at night

This is unusual in the school-age child because sleep is particularly sound between about 5 years of age and puberty. However, sleep might be interrupted by *parasomnias* in which the child wakes up (e.g. nightmares). The parasomnias are discussed in chapter 6.

'*Growing pains*' at night have been said to be a cause of sleeping difficulties in otherwise healthy children, but the nature of this condition is obscure for lack of sufficient study. Typically, the child is either troubled at the end of the day or wakes at night complaining of leg pains which are eased by parental rubbing. The problem eventually resolves spontaneously. In the meantime, parents are usually reassured by the term 'growing pains' but, before making this diagnosis, it is important to exclude rheumatological and other physical illness to explain the symptoms (Atar et al., 1991). *Muscle cramps* at night are a common complaint, but the true nature of this entity is also ill-defined.

Early morning wakening

The whole family is likely to be affected if a child habitually wakes very early, does not go back to sleep and is noisy or demands attention. Inappropriately early feeds and napping early in the day were mentioned previously as reasons why infants might wake too early. In older children, there are other possible explanations.

- At this and any other age, sleep may be disturbed in the early morning by noise from outside the home, or within it from other members of the family. Early morning light can also disturb sleep. If this happens consistently, early waking becomes habitual. Steps need to be taken to ensure that the *sleeping environment* is conducive to sleep throughout the night. For example, blinds or curtains made from blackout material can be very useful.

- If the child is put to bed very early in the evening and readily goes to sleep he will wake in the early hours because by that time his sleep requirements have been met. In this '*advanced sleep phase syndrome*' the pattern of sleeping, waking and feeding is entirely normal except that the timing of the whole sequence is inappropriate. The child is ready for bed very early in the evening without any encouragement from his parents whose only concern is that he wakes up before they want him to do so. The aim of treatment is not to increase the child's total amount of sleep (which is usually not possible) but to delay bedtime (and other activities which provide time cues, especially mealtimes) by gradual steps, for example about 10 minutes each evening.

   As children grow up, they need less sleep. Because the time to start the day tends to remain the same to fit in with the family's general activities, bedtime usually becomes progressively later. Occasionally, an early bedtime is maintained over the years with the result that the child wakes very early when he has had enough sleep. The solution lies in changing the bedtime to a time that is more in keeping with the child's age.

CASE: A 10-year-old girl woke regularly at 5 a.m. mainly to the consternation of her parents because of the disturbance created by her attempts to entertain herself. Enquiries revealed that she still went to bed in the early evening (as she had done since she was small) because this was convenient for her parents (both of whom had worked night shifts for some years) and their child-minding arrangements. As she had become older, her sleep requirements had lessened to the point, at the time of referral to the sleep clinic, that she had obtained enough sleep by 5 o'clock in the morning.

By increasing her evening activities, it was possible to shift her sleep phase later by gradually delaying her bedtime eventually by about $2\frac{1}{2}$ hours as a result of which she began to wake spontaneously by about 7.30 a.m.

Comment: This case illustrates how parental shift work (which is increasingly more common) or other ways in which unusual domestic arrangements can adversely affect children's sleep patterns. It was also evident that the fact that their daughter's sleep requirements would change as she became older had not been appreciated by her parents.

- Just as early waking in infancy can be reinforced by early feeds, older children may become *conditioned* to wake early because they are able to indulge in pleasurable activities at this time (e.g. watching videos, eating). This was partly the problem in the case just described. Such activities should be discouraged in a way that avoids conflicts and resentment. Some parents find it useful to use visible signals (e.g. signs hung on the bedroom door-handle) to let the child know when it is acceptable to leave their room.
- If the explanations just considered have been explored and really do not apply, it may be that the child who wakes early needs less sleep than most of his age (so-called '*short sleeper*') or he may be constitutionally a '*lark*' as described earlier. If this is so, the potential for altering the child's sleep pattern will probably be limited. Adapting to the situation by whatever means suits the family will be necessary (e.g. by providing the child with a form of entertainment that does not disturb other people) until, hopefully, the situation improves with time.

Adolescence

High rates of serious sleep problems have been consistently reported in adolescents. This is generally thought to be mainly a consequence of the marked psychological and social changes associated with this stage of development. Before adolescence, bedtime and getting-up time are largely set by parents. Increasingly, during the teenage years, the adolescent acts independently in deciding when to go to bed and, to some extent, when to get up although this may be determined by early day activities such as travelling to school or college at a distance from home or, sometimes, by early morning employment.

Sleep complaints often take the form of a need for more sleep, but perhaps 15% describe difficulty falling asleep, staying asleep or waking too early (Morrison et al., 1992). The problems seem to increase over the teenage years with no definite differences between the sexes. Difficulty getting to sleep might be partly biologically based, with a tendency towards delay of the circadian sleep phase for the physiological reasons described in chapter 3.

The following possible causes of sleeplessness should be considered:

- *Worries and anxiety* about school, work, personal life or other sources of stress. Multiple sleep problems are particularly associated with high levels of psychological disturbance, especially anxiety and depression. Measures for dealing with worries at night were mentioned earlier.

- *Erratic sleep–wake schedules* (chapter 5). These are not confined to adolescence and can result from a generally disorganized way of life in families with young children. However, teenagers' inconsistent sleep habits (including late nights at weekends or during holidays) and naps later in the day are particularly liable to produce a breakdown of circadian sleep–wake rhythms. The sleep disturbance may be worsened by the excessive consumption of *caffeine-containing drinks*, *alcohol* or *nicotine*, or by the use of *illegal substances* including during the withdrawal phase. Stimulant abuse produces long periods awake (perhaps several days) interspersed with long periods of excessive sleepiness (Obermeyer & Benca, 1996).

- Difficulty getting to sleep is very often part of the '*delayed sleep phase syndrome*' (DSPS). Although the condition occurs at all ages, it is especially common in adolescence. It will be discussed in chapter 5 in relation to daytime sleepiness (the main complaint in DSPS) resulting from sleep requirements not being met on days when getting up for school or other early day activities is necessary. Difficulty falling asleep is also severe and often lasts until the early hours, irrespective of the time of going to bed. The insomnia, and the difficulty getting up in the morning, are essentially physiological in nature but are easily misinterpreted as 'difficult adolescent behaviour'. Concern about not getting sufficient sleep can add to the problem. The situation is also made worse if alcohol or other substances are used in an attempt to get to sleep, or stimulants to keep awake during the day.

- These various sleep disorders may in themselves lead to serious psychological problems, but, as in adults, sleep disturbance in general can be an early symptom of major *psychiatric illness*, such as depressive illness, eating disorders, schizophrenia and mania. The importance of early detection and the prospects of preventing worsening of the underlying psychiatric condition by prompt attention to sleep disturbance have been emphasized by Breslau et al. (1996).

Obviously, management varies with the nature of the sleeplessness and its cause. Improved sleep hygiene, alterations to sleep schedules, and other measures related to the sleep disturbance itself may well need to be combined with specific treatment for any underlying condition such as depression.

Sleeplessness: basic clinical approach to diagnosis

(see Table 7 for specific causes)

1 What is the exact nature of the problem when parents say their child does not sleep?
   • What form of sleeplessness (e.g. bedtime difficulties, night waking, early morning waking) and how often the problem arises?
   • A sleep diary will provide a more accurate account.
2 Are their expectations reasonable?
   • Do they need explanation of what is normal?
   • Do they have other problems which are distorting their view?
3 If the child's sleep pattern is abnormal, consider the underlying sleep disorder and treat it accordingly, rather than:
   • simply reassuring parents that it is a passing phase;
   • treating it purely symptomatically with medication.
4 For this and other types of sleep problem assess the child's sleep adequately including:
   • a sleep history;
   • review of the child's 24-hour sleep–wake pattern;
   • developmental and family histories;
   • review of physical and mental health.
5 Consider general factors which may apply at any age:
   • Do the parents handle the child's bedtime and general behaviour inappropriately?
   • Are there other family problems that affect the child's sleeping?
   • Are the sleeping circumstances unsatisfactory?
   • Are there other factors preventing satisfactory sleep (i.e. poor sleep hygiene)?
   • Does the child have a medical condition (including treatment) that affects sleep?
6 The correct diagnosis is usually possible primarily by means of careful clinical assessment. Polysomnography or other special investigations are rarely required.

Infancy

1 The child may be of a type who generally cries more than most (including in the evening) without any organic cause.

2 Frequent waking and only returning to sleep by being fed suggests that the waking has been conditioned by unnecessary frequent feeding at night.

3 Close relationship of sleeping and other problems with certain types of food suggests allergy.

Early childhood

1 The number and timing of daytime naps may be inappropriate.

2 Parental practices and the circumstances surrounding bedtime and waking during the night may be at fault.

- Is there no consistent relaxing bedtime routine?
- Is bedtime unreasonably early?
- Is bedtime and going to sleep associated with pleasant or unpleasant experiences in the child's mind?
- Does the child need his parents' presence to be able to go to sleep?
- Are the circumstances different when the child goes to sleep and when he wakes in the night?
- Do parents give in to their child's delaying tactics at bedtime or demands to be with them if he wakes during the night?
- Does the child readily settle to sleep or go back to sleep in the night with one person but not another (suggesting failure to set appropriate limits)?

Middle childhood

In addition to enquiring about the possible explanations why toddlers may not sleep well consider:

- overarousal from exciting or boisterous activity near bedtime;
- night-time fears;
- worries about family or school matters which may no longer exist but have set up a habit of not sleeping well;
- being put to bed too early causing difficulty getting to sleep or waking early when sufficient sleep has been obtained for the child's age;
- the child may be constitutionally unable to get to sleep until late (although other explanations should be considered first).

Adolescence

Some of the above reasons for not sleeping well may still apply but the following possibilities should also be explored:

- changes in life style causing erratic sleep wake patterns or delay in the timing of the sleep period (easily misinterpreted as 'difficult adolescent behaviour');
- excessive caffeine intake, alcohol, tobacco;
- use of illegal substances;
- psychiatric disorder.

5

Excessive sleepiness

General aspects

A particularly neglected problem

Anders et al. (1978) took doctors to task for not paying more attention to excessive sleepiness in children: 'The sleepy child has been ignored by physicians attracting medical attention only after daytime sleepiness had seriously impaired their education.' As mentioned earlier, this reproach has still not been heeded and the problem remains neglected, despite the evidence that it is common and the reasons for supposing that it is linked with various difficulties and dangers comparable to those described in sleepy adults (reduced work performance, accidents including car crashes, impaired social relationships and even major disasters) (Mitler, 1996).

There are a number of explanations why childhood sleepiness has not received the attention that it merits.

- Compared with the other main sleep problems of sleeplessness and the parasomnias, sleepiness is less obvious and also less troublesome. It may not be recognized as a problem until the child goes to school and has difficulty with school work or other activities.

- Even when the problem is acknowledged, the sleepy child may not come immediately to professional attention because the sleepiness is often not viewed as a medical problem by parents, teachers or children themselves. The symptoms are easily misinterpreted as laziness, awkwardness, boredom or poor motivation.

- If a professional opinion is sought, similar mistaken conclusions may be reached, or the sleepy behaviour viewed as a sign of depression or limited intelligence. Such mistakes seem particularly common in narcolepsy in which long delays in making the correct diagnosis often occur, as will be discussed later.

Excessively sleepy behaviour can vary widely according to a child's age, the degree of sleepiness and its pattern of occurrence.

Manifestations at different ages

Problems in correctly recognizing excessive sleepiness as such are increased by the fact that it can manifest itself differently according to the child's stage of development.

- Prolonged overnight sleep and naps may well be considered normal and desirable in a very young child rather than a cause of concern. Assuming they are aware of what is usual, parents are more likely to become anxious in the following circumstances:
  - if their child sleeps several hours longer than expected for a child of that age;
  - if napping continues beyond the age it would usually have ceased (e.g. after starting school);
  - if the child is sleepy at times when other children of the same age are active and alert;
  - if the child begins to sleep more than previously.
- The point has already been emphasized that, whereas sleepiness generally shows itself in adolescents and adults as a reduction or slowing of activities, in young children it can have the opposite effect, i.e. overactivity associated with poor concentration, irritability or aggression. Especially in young children, therefore, sleepiness and its cause should be considered routinely in any child with learning or behavioural problems.
- The naturally high level of daytime alertness in older prepubertal children may offset the excessive sleepiness at other ages in certain sleep disorders, such as obstructive sleep apnoea or narcolepsy. This masking effect is lost at adolescence when the tendency to sleep increases, as previously described.

Degrees of sleepiness

Sleepiness also varies in severity.

- At any age, the *mildly* sleepy person finds it difficult to make an effort or to concentrate for long periods, and may be irritable and generally out of sorts. Repeated yawning and stretching, drooping of the eyelids, eye rubbing, head nodding and general slowness may occur but without actually falling asleep other than at the right time and in an appropriate place.
- The *moderately* sleepy person may show some of the same features but cannot remain awake in comfortable circumstances which are conducive to sleep, for example when sitting reading or watching TV in a warm or darkened room, or when travelling as a passenger in a car.

- A *severe* degree of sleepiness occurs if the person falls sleep when doing something active such as eating, talking or walking about.

For everyday purposes, degree of sleepiness is best assessed in these clinical terms, including information from parents and teachers, possibly supplemented by a sleepiness scale as described in chapter 3. More detailed and objective assessment of sleepiness may be appropriate by means of the multiple sleep latency test (MSLT) in the diagnosis of certain causes of excessive sleepiness as described shortly.

Patterns of occurrence

The following patterns of occurrence of sleepy behaviour can be distinguished:
- continuous sleepiness during the day;
- discrete 'sleep attacks' (characteristically seen in narcolepsy);
- prolonged overnight sleep;
- intermittent excessive sleepiness rather than the more usual persistent form (see later).

'Hypersomnia' may be used to mean the same as excessive daytime sleepiness (EDS) or, more specifically, for unusually long periods of continuous sleep or excessively deep sleep.

Other manifestations of excessive sleepiness or related behaviour

The following states are described in adults. How often they occur in younger people is uncertain.
- *Automatic behaviour*: inappropriate and possibly complicated behaviour (often repetitive and meaningless) in a sleepy person with impaired registration of events and, therefore, amnesia for the period which may last from minutes to hours. Repeated 'microsleeps' (rapid alternation between wakefulness and sleep) may be responsible for such behaviour.
- *Sleep drunkenness*: inability to wake up fully for a long time after waking during which time the person is drowsy, disorientated, unsteady and may display automatic behaviour.
- *Subwakefulness*: not being able to stay alert during the day but without objective evidence of abnormal sleep at night or severe sleep abnormality during the day. There may be PSG evidence of drowsiness, however.

Sleepiness and other states of underactivity

Just as the meaning of 'sleeplessness' needs to be clarified, it is essential to establish exactly what is meant if a child is said to be very sleepy or tired.

'*Tiredness*' refers to a number of different conditions each likely to have different causes. '*Physical tiredness*' in the sense of lethargy, fatigue, exhaustion or lack of energy may well have a physical cause of which other signs are usually present. However, depressed people and, of course, people with the chronic fatigue syndrome complain of weariness or tiredness in this sense. A complaint of tiredness may also mean boredom or disinterest. '*Sleepy tiredness*' implies an urge to actually sleep showing itself in the different degrees of severity described earlier, either persistently or episodically.

As the distinction between 'sleepy tiredness' and 'physical tiredness' is not always easy to make (especially in children), the possibility of a physical cause for relative inactivity should always be considered by means of physical examination and also special investigations as appropriate. Anaemia and endocrine disorder are examples of possible medical causes of tiredness in general.

Occasionally, excessive sleepiness with long periods in bed is *simulated* in order to escape from a difficult situation. Detection of such cases requires careful observation and possibly physiological sleep studies.

CASE: For the previous 4 years a 14-year-old boy had intermittently spent long periods in bed at home for up to 20 hours at a time each day, only getting up for the toilet and for meals. These periods lasted 2–3 weeks at intervals of a few months. Investigations for a physical cause (including neuroimaging and basic EEG recordings) at various hospitals had all been normal. The possibility of the Kleine–Levin syndrome and treatment with stimulant drugs had recently been considered.

The same pattern continued when he started boarding-school where he was admitted to the school medical centre during his sleepy periods. Here the staff were able to observe him closely but unobtrusively and suspected that he was not actually asleep for most of the time in bed. Polysomnography (by means of a portable system) during these sleepy periods confirmed that he slept on average about 10 hours each night, the rest of the time being spent awake but relatively inactive, for example reading.

Enquiries eventually revealed much tension between the boy and his parents who had unrealistically high academic expectations which he was unable to fulfil. It then became clear that the prolonged episodes of staying in bed apparently asleep were consistently related to the prospect of examinations or some other challenge which he had come to expect would be a further cause of embarrassment to himself and disappointment to his parents.

Treatment was suggested aimed at reducing the boy's need to opt out of difficult situations by improving his relationship with his parents but this was refused. Some months later the parents reported that their son had been 'completely cured following a single visit to a hypnotherapist'!

Comment: The psychological setting of sleep problems is generally important. Ignoring family factors in such a case as this would obviously lead to misinterpretation of the nature and origins of the sleep problem and to inappropriate advice. The solution to such complex family issues can be difficult. Perhaps in this case the apparent success of hypnotherapy represented at least a temporary solution to the boy's difficulty based on finally confronting the problem and changing his behaviour without loss of face.

Table 9. Differential diagnosis of excessive sleepiness in older children and adolescents

Insufficient sleep (including circadian sleep–wake cycle disorders)
  Insomnia
  Late night activities combined with getting up early
  Irregular sleep–wake schedule
  Delayed sleep phase syndrome
  Non-24 hour sleep–wake syndrome

Disturbed sleep
  Recreational drugs (caffeine, alcohol, nicotine)
  Illicit drugs, including withdrawal
  Medical and psychiatric disorders
  Medication
  Upper airway obstruction
  Other sleep disorders (frequent parasomnias, periodic limb movements)

Increased need for sleep
  Narcolepsy
  Idiopathic CNS hypersomnia
  Depression
  Neurological disease
  Other physical illness
  Congenital long sleeper
  Kleine–Levin syndrome (intermittent sleepiness)
  Menstruation-related hypersomnia (intermittent sleepiness)

Prevalence and causes of excessive sleepiness

As many as 5% and possibly more of the young adult male population are thought to suffer from excessive sleepiness (Billiard et al., 1987). The figure for children is not known, but it must be quite high in view of the many conditions of which sleepiness is a feature and which collectively are common. Adolescence is a particularly vulnerable period for the development of excessive sleepiness and its adverse effects such as academic underperformance, impaired social relationships, low mood and possibly accidents and other mishaps. When asked, perhaps the majority of adolescents feel in need of more sleep than they usually obtain and this complaint is associated with self-reports of low mood and underfunctioning (Wolfson & Carskadon, 1998). However, younger children are by no means exempt from excessive sleepiness in its various forms.

The many conditions and circumstances causing excessive sleepiness are listed in Table 9. They are grouped as:

- insufficient sleep, including circadian sleep–wake cycle disorders;
- conditions in which sleep is disturbed, affecting its quality and restorative value;
- disorders in which sleep requirements are pathologically increased.

Insufficient sleep including circadian rhythm disorders

Chronic lack of sleep

This is a common cause of excessive daytime sleepiness. The various reasons (discussed in the previous chapter) why the number of hours of overnight sleep (or, in the case of young children who normally nap during the day, total sleep each 24-hour period) might be persistently reduced need to be considered. Insufficient sleep and disturbed circadian sleep–wake rhythms are generally thought to be the main cause of excessive sleepiness in adolescence in particular, worsening as this phase of development proceeds. The use of alcohol, tobacco and coffee may well add to this effect (Tynjälä et al., 1997).

It is generally considered that the combination of late-night social activities, staying up late for study but having to get up early for school or early morning activities (e.g. newspaper delivery round) reduces the number of hours many older children and adolescents sleep to below that needed for satisfactory daytime functioning (the '*adolescent sleep debt*'). As discussed already, the risk of problems arising is increased at puberty when physiological sleep requirements do not decrease as they do progressively at earlier ages and the sleep phase tends to become delayed. Difficulty getting off to sleep at night and recurrent waking make the problem worse, or may be sufficient in themselves to reduce or seriously impair sleep. The result is considerable difficulty getting up in the morning, irritability, emotional lability, lethargy or actually falling asleep during the day, perhaps especially in the afternoon. Inadequate sleep is suggested by sleeping much longer when the opportunity arises at weekends or during holidays. The pattern of significantly less sleep on school nights than at the weekend is said to be characteristically adolescent (Szymczak et al., 1993).

Identification of this state of affairs requires careful enquiries to the individual and other members of the family about sleep–wake and other schedules both during the week and at weekends. A sleep diary over 2–3 weeks can be very valuable compared with generalizations about 'usual' sleep habits and patterns.

Correction of the problem of late-night social activities requires a change of life style or other measures which may be difficult to achieve without there being strong motivation to do so. The ideal solution is an agreed, co-operative effort on the part of both the young person and his parents. Explaining the potentially serious effects of chronic lack of sleep sometimes provides the necessary incentive.

Circadian sleep–wake cycle disorders

Other measures will be needed if the habit of not going to bed late has developed into a disturbance of the circadian sleep–wake cycle. This may take the form of irregular sleep–wake schedules or the delayed sleep phase syndrome (DSPS).

Irregular sleep–wake schedule

Disorganized and variable sleep and waking behaviour was described earlier. This can occur at any stage in childhood as a result of lack of consistency and routine in family functioning. However, in adolescence additional influences may have the same effect, or make a pre-existing problem worse. Such factors as irregular mealtimes, inconsistent late-night social activities, variable times of going to bed and waking up, sleep disturbance caused by stress, and use of recreational and even illicit drugs may combine to disrupt basic circadian rhythms. The result may be loss of a clear sleep–wake rhythm with difficulty in getting off to sleep, staying asleep or confining sleep to night-time. Sleep is likely to be broken into a number of blocks, possibly of different duration, each 24 hours. The likely adverse effects were mentioned earlier, including underperformance at school or work, impaired social relationships, mishaps, low mood and unsociable behaviour.

The potential difficulty of correcting this situation should not be under-estimated. Education about the importance of regular sleep, and consistency and moderation in other activities, is important combined with attention to specific causes such as estrangement between the young person and his parents, or psychiatric disorder.

Delayed sleep phase syndrome (DSPS): general

This condition is common at all ages especially, it seems, at adolescence (Thorpy et al., 1988). As described in chapter 3, to maintain a regular daily sleep–wake cycle of 24 hours, entrainment by means of various time cues has to occur consistently. Without a regular schedule of activities at the right times, the sleep phase becomes delayed with the result that it is physiologically impossible to go to sleep earlier by choice, in spite of feeling tired and having been awake for a long time. Entreaties by parents to go to bed at a sensible time are ineffective. Likewise, getting up to go to school, for example, is very difficult because sleep requirements have not been met by that time. The sleep problems in DSPS, therefore, are a combination of difficulty getting off to sleep (as mentioned in chapter 4), and (especially) considerable difficulty getting up in the morning and staying awake during the day. In DSPS (and the advanced sleep phase syndrome also mentioned in the previous chapter) the abnormality lies only in the timing of sleep rather than its intrinsic nature.

Young children may develop the habit of going to bed late because of the kind of delaying tactics described earlier in relation to settling difficulties. Sometimes, parents keep their child up until late for company, or he may be kept awake until late by other children in the family with sleep problems of their own. Whatever the reason, the habit of going to sleep late becomes an inability to do otherwise. This results in confrontation and more serious struggles when parents want their child to go to sleep at a reasonable time.

Many *adolescents* develop their habit of staying up late because of late-night social or other recreational activities, or because of studying late. Coffee consumption and smoking in the evening adds to the problem. Staying up late is often combined with sleeping in late and perhaps taking an afternoon nap. Although the problem of not being able to get to sleep earlier may be the adolescent's main complaint, the more usual concern at this stage of development is inability to get up in the morning on weekdays and to function effectively during the day.

Diagnostic features of DSPS

The characteristic clinical features of DSPS about which specific enquiries should be made are:

- persistently severe difficulty getting to sleep;
- uninterrupted sound sleep once asleep;
- considerable difficulty getting up for school or work;
- sleepiness and underfunctioning especially in the morning and afternoon, giving way to alertness in the evening and early hours;
- sleeping in very late when able to do so at weekends and holidays (which maintains the sleep phase delay).

Information on these points may be obtained by means of a sleep diary kept over a 2–3 week period including questions directed at these aspects of the sleep–wake pattern. Actometry over a similar period is a valuable way of describing the sleep schedule objectively, especially if there is doubt about the accuracy of the clinical information or difficulty obtaining it.

Treatment of DSPS

This can be difficult partly because depression or other psychological difficulties commonly complicate the situation (Regestein & Monk, 1995). However, a determined attempt is needed because of the serious consequences of the condition.

Chronotherapy consists of progressively changing the sleep phase to an appropriate time (Czeisler et al., 1981). It is generally considered that how this is achieved depends on the severity of the sleep phase delay (Sheldon et al., 1992).

If the *delay is about 3 hours or less* the steps are as follows:

- For 1–2 days the child is allowed to go to sleep and get up at the times he is able to do so readily. In young children this should eliminate the bedtime struggles to everyone's relief.
- Waking up time is brought forward by about 15 minutes for a few days, keeping to the same bedtime. If, on most weekdays, the child is already getting up (albeit with difficulty) at the appropriate time to go to school on time, it is not necessary to bring the waking time forward in this way, but it is important that

he is woken up and actually gets up at the same time at weekends and during holidays.

- For the last few days of this stage, bedtime is brought forward by about 15 minutes each night for several nights.
- When the child is effectively sleep deprived (making it easy to go to sleep), the waking-up time should continue to be brought forward as before.
- When a bedtime has been achieved such that the child goes to sleep promptly, bedtime should then be firmly fixed, ensuring that the total sleep period is appropriate for the child's age and adequate for him to be able to get up in the morning without difficulty.

Obviously, during part of this sequence the child will be short of sleep and co-operation may be difficult. He may also want to sleep during the day but this must be resisted. Families are likely to need professional help in seeing through this programme over the several weeks that it lasts.

CASE: An 11-year-old girl was reported as having difficulty getting to sleep at night associated with daytime sleepiness for over a year. On enquiry, it was apparent that her parents asked her to go to bed at 9 p.m. but she would resist going, asking to watch more TV and saying that she was not tired. After arguments she eventually went to her room where she read in bed until she fell asleep, usually about midnight. She then slept soundly but her parents had great difficulty waking her about 7.30 a.m. to go to school. At weekends she went to bed about 10 p.m. and she fell asleep at much the same time. She was then allowed to sleep in to catch up on 'lost sleep' and woke spontaneously about 10 a.m.

The girl was keen to change her sleep pattern because she was 'bored' when she could not fall asleep at night and disliked feeling tired at school, especially as she was keen to do well in her lessons.

Treatment for this delayed sleep phase involved several steps.

First, for a week she was allowed to go to bed when she wanted to (and not before 11 p.m.) so that all the family tension surrounding bedtime could be eliminated. The girl chose to go to bed about 11.45 p.m. and still fell asleep about midnight. At this time, because she was already being woken up at a suitable time on weekdays, it was not appropriate to have her wake up any earlier. Instead, her parents were asked to wake her at this time every morning, including weekends, and not allow her these 'catch-up' sleeps at the weekend. This made her somewhat more sleepy during the day.

Second, her bedtime was brought forward by about 15 minutes every other day. Because she was even more sleepy than usual, and now associated bed with sleep (rather than with family arguments and tension) she was able to adjust to this gradual change in her bedtime. Over the course of just over a week they managed to bring her bedtime to 10.45 p.m. after which she fell asleep within about 15 minutes without any difficulty.

She then attended a family party and went to bed later than usual. This disrupted the programme and they found that afterwards she was unable to go to sleep until about

11 p.m. The family were instructed to repeat the treatment programme as before, putting her to bed about 11.15 p.m. (15 minutes before she usually fell asleep), then 11 p.m., then 10.45 p.m. etc., and to make sure that these times were adhered to rigidly. Within 2 weeks they had reached a bedtime of 9 p.m. (more suitable for a girl of her age), she was falling asleep by 9.45 p.m. and then sleeping soundly until morning when she woke, often spontaneously, by 7.30 a.m.

She also kept to these bedtimes and wake-up times at the weekends. During the long school holidays, the parents let her go to bed 1 hour later (and to get up 1 hour later) but they were now able to retrain her body clock back to an appropriate time before the school term started again.

Comment: Providing both child and parents are motivated, quite long-standing sleep patterns can be changed by this type of systematic approach and setbacks dealt with satisfactorily. Explanation of the nature and purpose of the treatment (and assurance that it can work) before the programme is started are essential to maintain the family's efforts.

The need for professional support and encouragement is probably even greater to sustain the 'around the clock' treatment needed when the *sleep phase delay exceeds 3–4 hours*, as may well be the case in adolescence when it may be impossible to sleep until 4 a.m. or thereabouts. This form of treatment has the advantage of taking not more than several days. However, it needs to be carefully arranged because of its disruptive effects on the family as a whole, at one stage involving a complete reversal of normal sleep–wake patterns. The steps consist of:

- identifying typical sleep onset time, as above, allowing the child to go to sleep at this time and to sleep for as long as he needs;
- then progressively delaying bedtime by 2–3 hour steps each night (which will be followed by a similar delay in waking up time);
- once the described timing of the sleep phase is reached, wake-up time and bedtime must be firmly and consistently fixed each day including weekends and holidays.

Other aspects of management are as follows:

- The sleep phase advancing properties of *bright natural or artificial light* (Chesson et al., 1999a) after waking in the morning can be used to augment the above programmes. High intensity light boxes may be useful for the older child or adolescent.
- At this and other ages, attempts to change the timing of sleep will be helped by ensuring an appropriate level of illumination. For example, long periods during the day in a darkened room watching TV will interfere with the retiming programme; delaying wake-up time will be difficult if the bedroom is very well lit in the early morning by daylight through uncurtained windows (Ferber, 1995).

- Sleep hygiene principles are also important.
- It is essential that the corrected sleep schedules are rigidly maintained after the course of treatment has been completed.
- A firm agreement to maintain the new sleep pattern of social activities and sleep should be sought.

Chronotherapy treatment requires considerable motivation and commitment on the part of both patient and other family members. In some cases, the child or adolescent is not motivated to change, preferring the late-night activities. Alternatively, there may be some other psychological reason for not making the effort required, including avoidance of school. This situation has been called the '*motivated sleep phase delay*' (Ferber & Boyle, 1983). Characteristically, attempts to treat the sleep problem meet with no enthusiasm or even resistance, and the timing of the sleep phase may become more normal when the prospect of these activities is more attractive, for example during holidays. An understanding of the patient's attitudes and family situation is needed to anticipate such complications and to establish the best way of dealing with them including psychiatric help, if necessary.

CASE: The parents of a 15-year-old boy were concerned that it was particularly difficult to get him up in the morning and that he often played truant, not arriving at school after he had left the house. His father left home very early each morning for work and his mother was also out all day at work. It eventually came to light that on the days that he truanted he returned home to sleep. For some time he had been in the habit of staying out late in the evenings with his friends before returning home and going straight to his bedroom to watch TV or listen to music until the early hours. Typically he got to sleep between 1 and 2 a.m. During a recent holiday in the USA, the boy's sleep pattern had returned to normal with no difficulty getting up in the morning, but soon after return to the UK he reverted to his usual sleep–wake pattern.

On the basis of this story, and further information from a sleep diary kept over a 3-week period, a diagnosis was made of the delayed sleep phase syndrome which had been temporarily corrected by the time-zone difference when he was on holiday.

Gradual advancement of his sleep phase met with only temporary success in spite of his apparent effort to comply with treatment. Following complete relapse, further enquiries revealed a serious long-standing antagonism between the boy and his father whose company in the evenings he had come to avoid by staying out late and pre-occupying himself in the seclusion of his bedroom. Considerable effort was required before their relationship was improved. Reintroduction of the chronotherapy was then followed by a sustained improvement in the boy's sleep pattern.

Comment: Especially in such a case as this, it is important to take a comprehensive view of the child's psychological state and the family situation. This is more likely to be effective than applying chronotherapeutic measures in a mechanical fashion.

Melatonin has been heralded as a valuable and uncomplicated treatment for various sleep–wake cycle disorders, but these expectations have not always been fulfilled in children (Jan et al., 1999b). The uncertainties of melatonin as a therapeutic agent were considered in chapter 3.

Although supposedly common, DSPS is not well known by professionals or the public. As a result, it is particularly likely to be misconstrued as troublesome 'teenage' behaviour.

CASE: The mother of a 15-year-old girl had been convicted because of her daughter's erratic attendance at school over the previous 12 months. Mother appealed against the conviction on the grounds that her daughter had a sleep disorder as distinct from dislike of school to which the school authorities had attributed her failure to get up for school on time.

When a sleep history was taken it was evident that over the past 3 years she had been going to sleep progressively later because of reading, watching television or doing homework in her bedroom until late at night. She usually drank at least two mugs of coffee during these activities. When seen in the sleep clinic she had reached the point of going to her room about 10 p.m. but was unable to sleep until 2–3 a.m. after which she slept soundly. Her mother's attempts to wake her at 8 a.m. for school were strongly resisted and increasingly she would go back to sleep and either not go to school at all or arrive there late.

On the days she attended school, the girl described herself as 'feeling terrible'; others described her as 'looking awful' and 'very morose'. Sometimes she had actually fallen asleep at school. By evening she had become reasonably alert again. At weekends and during school holidays she still had difficulty getting to sleep until the early hours of the morning, but was in the habit of catching up on her sleep by sleeping in until late morning or early afternoon. The patient was of above average intelligence and keen to succeed academically.

It was considered that she displayed classic features of the delayed sleep phase syndrome with chronic sleep loss. There was no evidence that she was trying to avoid school. This interpretation was accepted by the court and her mother's conviction was then quashed. A treatment programme, based on a detailed diary description of the girl's sleep pattern, was devised involving progressive sleep phase delay which the girl and her family carried out with determination. She soon became able to go to sleep by around midnight and had much less difficulty getting up in the morning.

Comment: This is just one example of how the behaviour of someone with a sleep disorder can be misjudged because of the general lack of knowledge (in this case mainly by the education authorities) of sleep disorders and their possibly serious effects on behaviour.

Non-24 hour sleep–wake syndrome (entrainment failure)

This form of circadian sleep–wake abnormality is much less common than the irregular type or DSPS. It is essentially the result of failure to entrain to a 24-hour period, i.e. to advance the sleep phase each night. This can result from damage to the brain pacemaker mechanisms controlling sleep and wakefulness, as in children with widespread cerebral damage or maldevelopment (usually associated with severe learning disability), or from localized hypothalamic dysfunction.

Alternatively, blindness is the cause because of the absence of light perception as a zeitgeber for the entrainment of endogenous sleep–wake rhythms as discussed in chapter 3.

As the tendency in these circumstances to fall asleep slips later by about one hour each night, a main complaint is increasing sleeplessness. There is also a need to sleep in later and later each morning. This causes increasing daytime sleepiness (and its consequences for daytime functioning) if the child has to get up at a set time. The sleep period gradually works its way around the clock so that there is a temporary phase in which the normal sleep–wake timing is reversed, and then later a phase when the child's sleep pattern is normal before the cycle repeats itself. Often the sleep–wake pattern is complicated by the disruptive effects of the psychological consequences within a family of the child's highly abnormal sleep.

Treatment can be difficult. The main aim is to boost environmental cues to entrainment, combined with very regular bedtimes and wake times, as well as firmly fixing the timing of other daily events including mealtimes and social activities.

Disturbed overnight sleep

General factors

If the sleep–wake pattern appears to be satisfactory, ways in which sleep may be interrupted and its restorative quality reduced have to be considered. Disruptive influences include:

- caffeine-containing drinks (notably coffee and cola drinks);
- tobacco and alcohol;
- frequent parasomnias;
- medical conditions such as nocturnal asthma or epilepsy;
- medication including hypnotic and sedative drugs (due to inadequate dosage or rebound effects);
- illicit drugs, including withdrawal effects.

CASE: A 16-year-old girl was referred to the sleep disorders clinic with only a 12-month history of difficulty getting off to sleep and recurrent night waking. During the same period she had also complained of tiredness, poor concentration and headaches sufficient for her to stop attending school. There was a history of a throat infection preceding these symptoms, but otherwise she had always been healthy with no worries about school and no other psychological problems. Extensive physical investigation had revealed no abnormality. A diagnosis of the chronic fatigue syndrome had been made and treatment had consisted of a small dose of imipramine at night, partly to help her to sleep but also because she was thought to be moderately depressed about the effect of her condition on her education.

On review, she denied using alcohol, tobacco or illicit drugs and there was no evidence of physical or serious psychiatric disorder. The only finding relevant to her sleep problems (apart from her emotional state which appeared to be a consequence of her other symptoms) was that for the last year she was in the habit of drinking large amounts of Coca Cola especially in the early evening because she felt thirsty and preferred this to other drinks.

She was initially reluctant to change this habit, but was eventually persuaded and converted to drinking only moderate amounts of a noncaffeine-containing soft drink instead. Within 2 weeks her sleep improved and also her depressive feelings without the need for the psychiatric intervention that had previously been planned.

Comment: This was an apparently very satisfactory response to a simple measure. However, follow up is important to see if the situation proves to be more complicated than it seemed, as might well be expected during adolescence.

Sleep disruption is also a main effect in the following primary sleep disorders.

Periodic limb movements and restless legs syndrome (Trenkwalder et al., 1996)

Periodic limb movements in sleep (PLMS) are brief and stereotyped contractions (usually about 2 seconds in duration) mainly affecting the toes, knees and hips, typically at intervals of about 20–40 seconds. They usually occur in NREM sleep with or without PSG evidence of arousal. Their severity is expressed as the number of movements (with or without arousals) per hour (PLM index or PLM arousal index). *Periodic limb movement disorder* (PLMD) is diagnosed if the rate exceeds 5 per hour with clinical evidence of sleep disruption or excessive daytime sleepiness.

PLMD has been viewed as a cause of excessive daytime sleepiness in adults (because of the fragmentation of sleep caused by repeated arousals) either as a cause in its own right, or as a contributory factor in other sleep disorders with which it may coexist, such as OSA or narcolepsy. However, doubt has been expressed recently about the association between PLMS and excessive sleepiness (and insomnia) other than when it is attributable to OSA or narcolepsy in which (like REM sleep behaviour disorder, discussed in chapter 6) PLMS are prominent. It is suggested that PLMS are related to impairment of dopaminergic systems (Montplaisir et al., 2000). PLMD can also be associated with various metabolic disorders, the use of antidepressants, or the withdrawal of various other drugs which act on the central nervous system. Detection of PLMS involves anterior tibialis and arousal monitoring as part of extended PSG.

PLMS may be accompanied by the *restless legs syndrome* (RLS) in which there is difficulty going to sleep because of disagreeable leg sensations, with an irresistible urge to move the legs. The condition can be very distressing. It is sometimes associated with physical illness such as uraemia. Most people with RLS also have PLMS.

Both PLMS and RLS have conventionally being considered rare in children and adolescents but recent reports suggest otherwise. PLMS in particular has been implicated as a cause of daytime ADHD symptoms, supposedly as a result of insufficient or poor-quality sleep, which improve with treatment including the use of dopaminergic medication (Picchietti & Walters, 1999; Picchietti et al., 1999). Reference was made earlier to the report of PLMS in children with Williams syndrome whose sleep improved in response to clonazepam (Arens et al., 1998).

Detection rests on enquiries about jerking movements during sleep and unpleasant leg sensations at night (sometimes regarded in children as 'growing pains' (see chapter 4)), with PSG for full evaluation of PLMS. PLMS should be differentiated from sleep starts and myoclonic seizures. Conditions somewhat clinically similar to RLS include muscle cramps, peripheral neuropathies and certain muscle disorders.

Response to various reported treatments (best confined to those with sleeplessness or excessive sleepiness convincingly caused by PLMD or RLS), such as dopaminergic agents, clonazepam, opioids, gabapentin and clonidine, seems to be variable in adults (Chesson et al., 1999b). In the absence of information about specific treatment in young patients, emphasis is placed on good sleep hygiene (perhaps especially caffeine restriction) although medication may be justified in some cases.

Upper airway obstruction (UAO): obstructive sleep apnoea (OSA) and the upper airway resistance syndrome (UARS)

Osler's 1892 account of chronic tonsillitis includes a detailed account of OSA in children, caused by enlargement of the tonsils and/or adenoids. Osler was insistent that 'parents should be frankly told that the affection is serious, one which impairs the mental not less the bodily development of the child'. He was of the opinion that: 'In spite of the thorough ventilation of this subject by specialists, practitioners do not appear to have grasped as yet the full importance of this disease. They are far too apt to temporize and to postpone unnecessarily medical measures' (Osler, 1892).

This may still be the case, despite the fact that OSA is the best-documented form of sleep-disordered breathing. Detailed descriptions (including the uncertainties about childhood OSA) are available from centres where a special interest has been taken in children with the condition (e.g. Carroll, 1996; Kirk et al., 1998). The following account is confined to main points of importance for the nonspecialist.

Terminology

Terminology can be confusing, especially as 'OSA' is sometimes used in children to include obstructive breathing problems during sleep without actual apnoeic episodes. The inclusive term *upper airway obstruction (UAO)* will be used here to cover the range of related conditions in which breathing is compromised during sleep by obstruction of the upper airway, as distinct from compromised respiratory function at a lower level, for example in asthma.

Apnoea can be central or obstructive and the two may coexist (*mixed apnoea*). *Apnoeas of prematurity or infancy* are usually central in origin and benign, reflecting the usual instability of the control of breathing at this stage of development. Indeed, periodic breathing in infancy is normal. Pathological forms of early apnoea, including congenital central hypoventilation syndrome ('Ondine's curse'), and their consequences have been discussed by Gaultier (1999).

In *central apnoea* there is no effort to breathe because brainstem respiratory mechanisms are affected, as in some brain-damaged children. However, in pure central apnoea, even with very infrequent breathing, neither the child nor the parent may be aware of the abnormality unless a change in the child's colour is observed. In *mixed apnoea*, such as that often seen with viral infections, the child may wake at night gasping or choking and may be cyanosed or pale. If the episodes are frequent, daytime symptoms are similar to those seen in OSA.

Obstructive apnoea implies interruption of airflow at the nose and mouth in spite of respiratory effort, because of obstruction of the airway. Chronic noisy breathing, including snoring, is the main sign of upper-airway obstruction and is caused by vibration of soft tissue structures as air is drawn in forcefully to overcome the obstruction.

Snoring to some degree occurs in perhaps 10% of children. A distinction has been made between *primary snoring* (PS), accounting for about 80% of all snoring children and not associated with sleep disruption or daytime symptoms, and the rest who have OSA causing a disturbance of the child's sleep physiology and clinical condition (Carroll & Loughlin, 1995a). In fact, this clear-cut distinction is being replaced by the view that there is continuum of sleep-related upper-airway obstruction ranging from a minimal degree of partial obstruction (causing primary snoring) to the other extreme of complete obstruction producing the full OSA syndrome. It is suggested that between these extremes there are other degrees of partial obstruction, i.e. the '*upper-airway resistance syndrome*' or *UARS* (Downey et al., 1993). It is possible that in some children the degree of obstruction, and its consequences, increase during the course of development.

The adverse effects on daytime functioning may also vary, the lesser degrees of airway obstruction causing less dramatic but yet significant harm. For example, it has been reported that snoring in general is associated in medical students in doing less well in examinations (Ficker et al., 1999).

Because history alone is thought to be unreliable in distinguishing different degrees of UAO or, indeed, primary snoring (Carroll et al., 1995), careful PSG evaluation of any child with chronic noisy breathing (including snoring) is, in principle, appropriate. In actual practice, this is difficult to achieve in view of the numbers involved and availability of resources.

UARS may be more common than OSA but has received less attention. An increase in respiratory effort can compensate for lesser degrees, but above a certain level sleep is sufficiently fragmented by arousals that clinical symptoms similar to OSA are caused. In the absence of the frequent apnoeas and hypopnoeas which characterize OSA on PSG, however, the extent of sleep disruption may not be appreciated and daytime symptoms not attributed to abnormal breathing during sleep.

Pathophysiology

Children with UAO usually have narrowing of their upper airway, but sometimes an abnormality of its neuromotor control (as in cerebral palsy), or weakness of upper-airway muscles, for example in spinal muscular dystrophy. During sleep, upper-airway tone is reduced. This predisposes to collapse and obstruction resulting in hypoxaemia and hypercapnia. Each time this happens (perhaps very many times), the child may arouse without actual wakening. However, as mentioned in chapter 3, such arousals are possibly less common in children than in adults with OSA, and with less overall disturbance of sleep architecture, including reduction of slow wave sleep.

Prevalence

The figures already quoted suggest that, in the general population, perhaps as many as about 2% of children from infancy onwards have some degree of sleep-related upper-airway obstruction. In the specially predisposed groups (such as those with a learning disability) the prevalence greatly exceeds this. Figures quoted for any of the forms of UAO may well be underestimates because of the lack of reliable epidemiological information. Such information is difficult to obtain because snoring may go undetected or it may be ignored, and there are, of course, inherent problems in undertaking large-scale physiological studies of respiratory function during sleep.

Predisposing factors (see also Stores & Wiggs, in press)

- In the general population, the main cause of UAO is *enlarged tonsils and adenoids*. However, there are many other possibilities to consider, but their absence does not exclude UAO, nor do any of them necessarily distinguish between OSA and UARS.
- As in adults, *obesity* is a predisposing factor, but only the minority of children with the condition are overweight and some may be quite the opposite, or have generally failed to thrive if the problem began very early in life.

- Other conditions which may reduce the calibre of the upper airway include *mucosal congestion, polyps, abnormalities of the soft palate, high-arched palate, large tongue, micro- or retro-gnathia,* and *upper-respiratory-tract infection.* UAO has been described in many *craniofacial syndromes,* such as Pierre-Robin syndrome, where there may be a number of structural abnormalities of the upper airway or related structures. Such craniofacial syndromes as Pfeiffer's or Crouzon's often have very severe UAO which is particularly difficult to treat. Guilleminault et al. (1996) have reported that children with a combination of mandibular abnormality (including a small triangular chin), palatal abnormality and long oval-shaped face are very likely to have some degree of UAO, although the absence of such features does not exclude this possibility.
- Reference was made earlier to the fact that UAO occurs widely in children with a *learning disability,* although this aspect of their predicament is often overlooked (Stores, 1992). The main example is *Down syndrome* in which a number of congenital abnormalities of the upper airway and related structures, together with possible obesity and hypotonia, may conspire to cause obstruction. In possibly the majority of children with this condition there is some degree of UAO during sleep which may impair their daytime psychological, and sometimes physical condition. However, it has been reported that the sleep of children with Down syndrome is often disrupted by frequent awakenings and arousals which are only partly related to UAO (Levanon et al., 1999). Other conditions in which OSA may be a prominent feature include the *mucopolysaccharidoses, fragile-X syndrome,* some cases of *Prader–Willi syndrome* and the various learning disability syndromes (often genetic in origin) which include craniofacial abnormalities.
- Other *neurological conditions* include some forms of *cerebral palsy, neuromuscular disease* (e.g. Duchenne muscular dystrophy or myotonic dystrophy), *spina bifida/myelomeningocele, hydrocephalus* and the *Arnold–Chiari malformation.*
- A predisposition to UAO is also seen in *achondroplasia, sickle cell disease* and other diseases in which upper-airway tissues may become infiltrated or impinged upon (e.g. by tumour).
- *General factors* which have been implicated are sedative medication, alcohol and passive smoking (Corbo et al., 1989). Allergies are associated with sleep disordered breathing but the mechanisms involved are not properly understood (McColley et al., 1997).

CASE: A 10-year-old boy with Down syndrome was assessed as part of a clinical research project. When a sleep history was taken, his mother reported that his sleep had been disturbed for as long as she could remember. She described his breathing as erratic and said he snored and made gasping and choking noises throughout the night which were loud enough to wake her and her husband. The child often slept with his head tipped back and was generally a very restless sleeper. Mother was particularly concerned that he repeatedly stopped breathing for periods of up to 30 seconds throughout the night as a result of which his parents felt it necessary to keep checking on him at frequent intervals. Both his mother and teachers described him as falling asleep repeatedly during the day and as being irritable and easily frustrated much of the time.

When for the first time she was informed about the high rate of OSA in children with Down syndrome, the boy's mother consulted his paediatrician, but the matter was not taken any further on the grounds that there was little that could be done in view of the child's basic condition.

Both night- and day-time problems worsened over the next few months and, following frequent requests by the child's mother, he was eventually referred to an ENT surgeon with a special interest in OSA. Overnight sleep studies revealed a severe degree of OSA which was attributed to congenital narrowing of the upper airway without evidence of adenotonsillar enlargement. Continuous positive airway pressure (CPAP) was successfully introduced despite the child's initial reluctance. Soon afterwards his mother reported that his breathing and his sleep at night were much improved and that he was more alert and manageable during the day.

Comment: The delay in recognizing OSA in this case might well be typical. In fact, this common problem in children with Down syndrome may not be identified at all, resulting in a lost opportunity to possibly improve the child's general well-being.

A report that breathing repeatedly stops should not necessarily be interpreted as evidence of central apnoea. If breathing noises stop, it might be thought that breathing itself must have stopped. It is important to encourage parents to look for chest and/or abdominal movements which, if they continue during the periods of interrupted breathing, indicate obstructive apnoea.

Presentation

As in other cases of excessive sleepiness, many cases of UAO will not come to light at all unless complications develop. Those that do come to professional attention may present in a number of ways depending somewhat on the age of the child. The same is true of narcolepsy, another important cause of excessive sleepiness discussed later.

Carroll & Loughlin (1995c) have provided a detailed review of the clinical features, including the various complications, that have been reported in children with UAO. There is more empirical support for some of these supposed features than for others. The variety of ways in which OSA may present include the following *general features*:

- *Abnormal sleepiness* (difficult to detect in young children) is more likely to be recognized at school age although it is easily misinterpreted as disinterest or daydreaming. Symptoms at this age may be particular difficulty waking up in the morning, perhaps with headache and bad mood, or daytime napping inappropriate for the child's age.

- The poor-quality sleep caused by UAO may cause various *behavioural problems*, including overactivity, poor concentration, impulsiveness or aggression. *School performance* may well deteriorate. Behavioural sleep problems may well coexist with the sleep disturbance caused by UAO (Owens et al., 1998).

The two main *specific signs* are:

- *chronic loud snoring* or other sounds of breathing difficulty during sleep, although absence should not be thought to exclude sleep disordered breathing if other suggestive features are present;
- *pauses in breathing or struggling to breathe* both of which can be particularly alarming for parents who may fear the child's life is at risk.

Other *suggestive features* are:

- recurrent *ear and throat infections*;
- *mouth breathing*;
- the *craniofacial abnormalities* described earlier.

Occasionally a child with UAO presents with one of the *complications* that have been associated with the condition.

- In young children UAO should be considered as a possible case of *failure to thrive* or a *decrease in growth rate*, as well as more *general developmental delay*.
- UAO has been implicated in some cases with *speech, eating or swallowing problems*, as well as *gastro-oesophageal reflux* and *pulmonary aspiration*.
- *Severe cardiovascular effects* (pulmonary hypertension, cor pulmonale) described in severe adult UAO are less likely in children other than those who have pre-existing heart defects, including some children with Down syndrome.
- Various *parasomnias* have been associated with UAO. Opinions differ about the link with *nocturnal enuresis*. *Sudden awakenings* with signs of distress are consistently reported in children with UAO at the end of an obstructive event, although their nature seems to be very variable. Some entail actual awakenings, with crying or moaning, others involve less dramatic movements or sounds of respiratory obstruction. *Nightmares* and *night terrors* have also been viewed as a complication of UAO for reasons that are unclear (Owens-Stively et al., 1996).

CASE: A 6-year-old girl was referred to the clinic from a child psychiatric service for advice on the management of nocturnal episodes which had convincing features of sleepwalking, sleep terrors and nightmares.

A screening sleep questionnaire completed by the family before attendance at the clinic, followed by a detailed sleep history (taken for the first time), revealed that for about the last 3 years she had always snored loudly. In addition, it came to light that her mother had observed her to stop breathing for short periods repeatedly during the night, that the child often slept with her neck extended and that she breathed through her mouth at night. She was particularly difficult to wake in the morning and, although not excessively sleepy during the day at school, she was described as overactive and making slow progress in learning to read and write. There was no early history of developmental delay and no family history of obvious relevance.

Further assessment confirmed the suspicion of upper-airway obstruction. Removal of her enlarged tonsils and adenoids was followed by resolution of her sleep disturbances (including the sleepwalking, sleep terrors and nightmares) and significant improvement in her behaviour and performance at school.

Comment: The case illustrates the tendency for a sleep history or even adequate screening not to form part of routine assessment in children's clinical services. The use of a screening questionnaire covering a range of possible sleep disorders can be a very useful screening device, even in busy paediatric or child psychiatry clinics.

Differences between UAO in adults and children (Marcus, 2000)

In recent years, awareness of UAO in adults has increased; less so in children. Awareness of the important differences between adults and children with the condition are important to avoid it being missed at an early age.

The typical adult with UAO is an obese middle-aged male who snores loudly, underfunctions during the day and responds to nasal continuous positive airway pressure treatment at night. This contrasts with the picture of childhood UAO in several ways, some of which have been mentioned already:

- most children are not obese (perhaps only 20%);
- the usual cause (or, at least, major contributory factor acting in combination with abnormal neuromuscular tone) is enlarged tonsils and/or adenoids, the removal of which often seems to be beneficial (although recurrence occurs in some cases);
- the sex ratio is equal;
- periods of partial airway obstruction with hypoventilation associated with hypercapnia ('*obstructive hypoventilation*') are often seen rather than the discrete, cyclical obstructive apnoeas in adults;
- sleep physiology is generally less disrupted;
- the behavioural consequences may be overactivity and other disruptive behaviour rather than obvious sleepiness during the day which is uncommon in children.

Assessment: general principles

The main *aims* of assessment are:

- to detect UAO and determine its severity;
- to exclude other causes of excessive sleepiness, or to identify any coexisting sleep disorder;
- to identify the causes of the obstruction, its associated features and any complications.

The guidelines to assessment suggested by Carroll & Loughlin (1995b) are as follows.

- A *provisional diagnosis* is possible from a *history* of chronic snoring or other signs of difficulty breathing during sleep, and the daytime and nighttime symptoms listed in Table 10. However, history alone does not clearly distinguish between PS, UARS and OSA.
- The usefulness of various *screening tests* remains the subject of debate. *Home audiovisual recordings* may clarify the description of breathing difficulties obtained in the clinic but a distinction between the different degrees of obstruction cannot necessarily be made. *Observation* of the child asleep and/or *overnight oximetry* are generally considered to be insufficiently sensitive procedures and a poor guide to severity. However, if overnight oximetry is abnormal, it indicates a severe degree of UAO; if the results are normal, lesser although possibly significant degrees of obstruction are not excluded (Brouillette et al., 2000).
- The prevailing view, in at least the USA, is that *diagnosis and assessment of the severity of* OSA requires *PSG* which also helps to identify or exclude other sleep disorders.
- Investigation of the *cause of the obstruction* by means of *fluoroscopy, endoscopy* or *radiological studies* is largely confined to children with craniofacial abnormalities.
- Detection of *complications* may involve *cardiological studies,* or *psychometric assessment* to assess the effects of the condition on daytime functioning.

As extensive investigation of all children who snore is not feasible, physiological sleep studies have to be used selectively. Reasonable indicators for *further investigation of children who snore* or who have some other form of chronic noisy breathing during sleep are:

- where parents describe their child stopping breathing at night or struggling to breathe during sleep;
- daytime somnolence or otherwise inexplicable behavioural disturbance;
- failing performance at school;
- very large tonsils or a clinical suggestion of enlarged adenoids;
- repeated upper-airway infection;
- poor growth rate or failure to thrive.

History

In addition to general history taking as discussed earlier, certain specific enquiries should be made if UAO is suspected.

Table 10 lists night-time and daytime features that may be evident in children with OSA in various combinations. The features listed are those commonly reported. However, the discriminating value of some of them is uncertain because

Table 10. Nighttime and daytime features of UAO

During sleep

Chronic loud snoring

Other sounds of breathing difficulty (gasping, snorting)

Other evidence of increased respiratory effort (retractions of chest-wall muscles, paradoxical inward movement of the chest during inspiration with outward movement of the abdomen)

Rapid breathing

Apnoeic episodes

Nasal flaring

Mouth breathing

Cyanosis

Unusual sleeping positions including kneeling or neck extension

Very restless sleep

Profuse sweating

Enuresis

Awakenings and associated parasomnias (night terrors, nightmares)

On waking

Difficulty waking up, disorientation, grogginess

Bad mood

Headache

Dry mouth

Daytime

Sleepiness

Concentration and memory problems, poor school progress

Irritability and other emotional or behavioural problems.

of limited information about their occurrence in the general population, their diagnostically nonspecific nature and also a shortage of controlled studies. The presence of some of the factors depends on the level of obstruction (e.g. at nasopharyngeal or oropharyngeal level), on the degree of the obstruction and, in some instances, the age of the child.

As in other cases of excessive sleepiness, the degree of sleepiness should be determined by clinical enquiry, possibly supplemented by the results of a sleepiness questionnaire such as the Epworth Sleepiness Scale adapted for use with children as mentioned in chapter 3.

Physical examination (Table 11)

This is directed to the nasal- and oro-pharynx, facial and cranial structures, and also general physical features.

Table 11. Main factors to consider on physical examination of child with UAO

Nasal obstruction
Congenital stenosis
Deviated septum
Nasal polyps
Foreign body
Rhinitis (seasonal or perennial)

Nasal- and oro-pharynx
Enlarged tonsils and adenoids
Large tongue
Abnormal hard palate inc. cleft-palate repair
Abnormal soft palate inc. abnormal uvula
Micrognathia

Craniofacial structures
Midface hypoplasia
Mandibular hypoplasia

General
Obesity
Adenoidal facies
Growth
Muscle tone
Evidence of neurodevelopmental syndromes (e.g. Down syndrome)
Chest, cardiac or neurological abnormalities

Physiological sleep studies

- As already stated, extended overnight PSG is usually recommended to establish the diagnosis of UAO in order to assess its type and severity and standards have been laid down for the investigation of this and other sleep-related breathing disorders (American Thoracic Society, 1996). PSG should be performed by a service skilled in working with children and their families (Loughlin et al., 1996). It is also important in evaluating the findings to acknowledge the differences in respiratory function between adults and children. Therefore, adult criteria are inappropriate (Rosen et al., 1992) and paediatric norms should be used (Marcus et al., 1992). PSG may need to be repeated if symptoms persist after treatment or if they recur.
- *Multiple sleep latency testing (MSLT)* to assess the degree of daytime sleepiness is not usually necessary unless the possibility of narcolepsy exists.

Treatment

The various medical and surgical treatments for UAO that have been reported have been the subject of little systematic evaluation. Similarly, the natural history and prognosis of OSA (whether treated or not) are not well known.

- The most usual treatment for children in the general population is combined *removal of tonsils and adenoids*. Because of possible postoperative complications, careful inpatient monitoring is recommended. Adenotonsillectomy may also be helpful in some children where the cause of the UAO is complex (e.g. those with Down syndrome) as the tonsils and adenoids may contribute critically to the obstruction without being obviously enlarged.
- CPAP or *bilevel positive airway pressure* (BiPAP) has been used successfully in children for whom removal of tonsils and adenoids is not appropriate or where it has not been effective. Again, a carefully considered approach, especially for children, is necessary for this procedure to be effective.
- *Weight reduction* is important for obese children with UAO.
- *More complicated surgery*, including uvulopalatopharyngoplasty (UPPP), has been reported in some cases of Down syndrome, cerebral palsy, craniofacial abnormalities and achondroplasia. *Tracheostomy* is viewed as a last resort and is rarely indicated.
- *Drug treatment* sometimes used in adults (such as tricyclic drugs), and *mechanical devices* aimed at reducing airway obstruction during sleep, appear to be ineffective in children.
- Medications for coexisting conditions which might depress respiration (notably benzodiazepines) should be avoided.

Conditions in which sleep tendency is increased

A need to sleep longer than normal and/or at times when it would be more normal to be awake is an intrinsic part of some conditions. This excessive sleepiness is usually persistent (as in narcolepsy) but can occur intermittently with normal sleep between the sleepy episodes (e.g. the Kleine–Levin syndrome).

Narcolepsy

CASE: A 14-year-old girl had been perfectly well until just 3 months before referral to the sleep clinic when she suddenly began to feel excessively sleepy most of the time. In addition, she began to have frequent short episodes of actually falling asleep including times at which she was engaged in various activities at home and at school. Within a week she reported experiencing brief slumping episodes, without loss of consciousness, when she was told jokes or suddenly alerted. About the same time she also described visual distortions of her bedroom and 'electric shocks' when drifting off to sleep sometimes accompanied by brief periods of not being able to move.

She became very frightened about going to bed because of the unpleasant nature of these experiences which soon began to occur every night. Her distress became worse when she also began to suffer from nightmares. Although she was unaware of their occurrence, her parents described further episodes characteristic of night terrors. Other troublesome experiences were occasional blurring of vision and double vision during the day.

There was no past personal or family history of significance. She was a previously happy and highly accomplished child. No abnormality was found on physical examination.

The clinical diagnosis of the narcolepsy syndrome was supported by overnight polysomnography including disrupted sleep and MSLT findings of a consistently short sleep latency (average 4.9 seconds) and REM sleep onset in 4 of the 5 opportunities to sleep.

Treatment was started consisting of methylphenidate and clomipramine combined with planned afternoon naps and advice about sleep hygiene. The nature of her condition was explained to all concerned, including her school teachers and peers. Within one month all her previous symptoms had resolved. A new feature of sometimes waking briefly several times a night (possibly a medication effect) was far less distressing than her earlier bedtime fears.

Comment: This case is unusual in the combination of sudden onset and rapid development of the full narcolepsy syndrome, prompt investigation and recognition of the condition, and quick and full response to treatment.

Prevalence

Narcolepsy (Bassetti & Aldrich, 2000) is a much misunderstood, often unrecognized and generally poorly managed condition. It is usually erroneously thought to be a rarity. Its estimated prevalence in the UK and the USA of 4–6 per 10,000 ranks it with much more readily acknowledged disorders such as Parkinson's disease and multiple sclerosis.

Onset

Age of onset is very variable with a reported range from 2 to over 60 years. However, in at least a third of cases (some suggest over 50%) the first symptoms appear in childhood or adolescence with an average onset at about 14 years of age. It has been reported that 16% of patients have had their first symptoms before 10 years of age and 4.5% before five years (Challamel et al., 1994). Unfortunately, a long delay is common before the correct diagnosis is made, often many years as in the series of children reported by Guilleminault & Pelayo (1998). Obviously such figures apply to those who come to medical attention; there is a fear that many cases do not reach this stage because the sleepiness in particular is not viewed as a medical problem.

Classical clinical features

The classical 'tetrad' of the full narcolepsy syndrome exemplified by the case just described is:

- Recurrent episodes of irresistible sleep (*sleep attacks*), lasting minutes to perhaps an hour and occurring in relaxed circumstances but also during various activities. Characteristically, these episodes of sleep are refreshing.
- Sudden loss of tone (*cataplexy*) for seconds or perhaps minutes, usually in response to strong emotion especially amusement or anger. Stress, fatigue or heavy meals, or even thinking of an amusing situation, have been reported to trigger attacks.
- Vivid and often terrifying dream-like experiences before falling asleep (*hypnagogic hallucinations*) or on waking (*hypnopompic hallucinations*).
- Episodes of inability to move when falling asleep or on waking (*sleep paralysis*). It may not be possible to speak or breathe properly as part of the attack, and there may be a fear of dying.

Each member of this classical tetrad can be viewed as a component part of REM sleep (i.e. sleep, atonia of the skeletal musculature, and dreaming) occurring separately and intruding into wakefulness. Therefore, narcolepsy appears to be mainly a disorder of REM sleep mechanisms, although there is also evidence of NREM sleep and possibly circadian sleep–wake rhythm abnormalities.

The usual sequence is for the sleep attacks to precede the appearance of the other symptoms, although all four symptoms eventually develop in less than 50% of cases. The approximate relative frequencies of the nonsleepiness ('ancillary') symptoms of the narcolepsy syndrome are:
- cataplexy: 100% where it is a requirement for a diagnosis of narcolepsy but others consider that cataplexy is not present in about 20% of cases;
- hypnagogic or hypnopompic hallucinations: up to about 50%;
- sleep paralysis: up to about 60%.

It should be remembered that *each of these ancillary symptoms can occur as an isolated phenomenon* (frequently, it seems, in the case of the hallucinatory phenomena and sleep paralysis) without being part of the narcolepsy syndrome.

In narcolepsy, *overnight sleep* is generally disrupted causing some degree of *persistent tiredness* during the day. Additional symptoms can include:
- *automatic behaviour*;
- *poor memory and concentration*;
- *visual disturbances*, such as blurred or double vision, of uncertain origin (the extraocular muscles are supposedly not involved in cataplexy).

There are ill-understood *associations* between narcolepsy and sleep apnoea, periodic limb movements in sleep and REM sleep behaviour disorder.

Aetiology

Genetic influences possibly of a multifactorial nature are prominent in narcolepsy, but environmental factors (such as inadequate or irregular sleep, psychological stress or physical illness) can precipitate episodes or can affect the severity of the condition at certain times. Recent research has demonstrated a deficiency of hypocretin (orexin) peptides in patients with the condition, raising the possibility of replacement therapy (Mignot, 2000).

It is usually thought rare for narcolepsy to be symptomatic of some other disorder, but associations have been described with various conditions in children including Niemann–Pick disease type C (Challamel et al., 1994). These authors suggest that the possibility of symptomatic narcolepsy should be seriously considered in preteenage children with narcolepsy, especially when cataplexy is very prominent (including status cataplecticus), where classical PSG findings are absent, or where human leucocyte antigen (HLA) typing is negative. However, it is doubtful whether some of the supposedly symptomatic cases should be classified as narcolepsy in the absence of the characteristic clinical and PSG features of the condition.

Special features of childhood narcolepsy (Stores, 1999a; Guilleminault & Pelayo, 2000)

As already stated, the condition very often begins at an early age. Because its effects on various aspects of development (cognitive, behavioural and social) can be very damaging, the long delays in its recognition and management are particularly serious.

The way in which narcolepsy first shows itself in children can be very different from the classical textbook descriptions of the disorder which tend to describe the symptoms in the fully developed adult form.

- In children the *sleepiness* may initially take the form of no more than prolonged overnight sleep which can be difficult to recognize in view of individual differences in sleep requirements. Indeed, as excessive sleepiness in general is hard to judge in young children, features other than obvious sleepiness are often the main initial complaint at that age (Guilleminault & Pelayo, 1998). The persistence of daytime naps after the age of about 4 is a more reliable sign of excessive sleepiness, but, as emphasized before, sleepiness in children can cause difficult behaviour, including overactivity.
- Although it is occasionally the initial symptom, the onset of *cataplexy* may be delayed many years or, according to some, it may not develop at all. Whenever it occurs, it may take a subtle form, such as buckling at the knees, drooping of the head or shoulders, arms dropping to the side, sagging of the jaw or merely a feeling of weakness or unsteadiness. Speech may become slurred or mouth movements unusual if muscle tone returns in bursts. Otherwise, limb movements may appear clumsy for the same reason.

Denial or concealment of these and other frightening or embarrassing aspects of narcolepsy (including hallucinations and sleep paralysis) can make recognition particularly difficult. Even when cataplexy is prominent, it may be misdiagnosed as a psychological condition, including conversion disorder (Dahl, 1996b). Other conditions with which cataplexy can be confused include seizures in which falling or collapse is the main feature (e.g. atonic or absences with loss of tone) or other 'drop attacks' of physical origin such as syncopal episodes, including those of cardiac origin. Important diagnostic features are that emotion (often laughter but also other positive as well as negative experiences such as fear) acts as a trigger, and eye and respiratory movements are preserved.

- Because of the nonspecific nature of the early features of narcolepsy, *other diagnostic errors* can occur including 'night terrors' in the case of very frightening hypnagogic hallucinations, or use of illicit drugs to explain the daytime sleepiness. Sometimes the child is thought to be limited intellectually.

- Especially in children, the symptoms of narcolepsy may be overshadowed by *secondary phenomena*. The case described earlier illustrates how night-time fears can develop, together with nightmares and sleep terrors. All these complications may dominate the picture if the actual narcolepsy features are less prominent than in that case. The sleepiness, embarrassment, misinterpretation of the symptoms and the restrictions imposed on educational, recreational and social activities, may all conspire to cause much distress. Depression, and the other psychological difficulties which are commonly described in children with narcolepsy (Kavey, 1992), easily lead to referral to educational or child psychiatric services without the basic nature of the condition being realized.

  It is important for child health and educational professionals to be aware that childhood narcolepsy is not a rarity and that it should be considered in any child who is sleepy, clumsy, has falling attacks or is psychologically disturbed.

Investigations

- PSG is indicated if narcolepsy is suggested, partly to exclude other causes of excessive sleepiness or other sleep disorders that can coexist with narcolepsy such as OSA or PLMD. At least in children age 8 and older, MSLT is appropriate (below this age the diagnosis has to rely mainly on the clinical history including elimination of other conditions as far as possible). However, the adult-based criteria for overnight PSG and MSLT have to be adjusted as prepubertal children (say between 8 and 11 years) are naturally very alert in the daytime. The mean sleep latency in children with narcolepsy may be less than about 10 minutes (rather than 5 minutes for adults) and some children do not initially show the two or more sleep onset REM periods (SOREMPs) out of the five MSLT naps seen in adult patients. As the adult physiological characteristics may not be evident until the condition has evolved, repeated assessment at intervals may be required.

- Human leucocyte antigen (HLA) typing is usually performed if narcolepsy is suspected. Type DQB1*0602 in particular is strongly associated with narcolepsy but its specificity is limited. A negative result makes the diagnosis unlikely, although some patients are described who are HLA negative and yet have the clinical features of narcolepsy (Parkes et al., 1998).
- Where the diagnosis of narcolepsy remains uncertain, it is important to regularly review the child's clinical condition and to repeat appropriate investigations at intervals as this might eventually reveal the diagnosis. However, failure to make a definite diagnosis does not necessarily remove the need for symptomatic treatment of the sleepiness.

Management

Narcolepsy is a lifelong condition which calls for particularly comprehensive and sustained care. In addition to medical aspects of the condition, educational, occupational, psychological and social issues must be considered in order to minimize possible adverse effects throughout life.

General aspects of management include:

- explanations to all concerned about the nature of narcolepsy, correcting in particular the idea that it is a character defect or other form of psychological disorder;
- advice about schooling, choice of career (avoiding occupations in which constant vigilance is essential), and other aspects of living such as driving regulations in the case of adolescents;
- promotion of sleep hygiene, including good sleep habits and routines;
- encouragement to lead an active and healthy life style (including avoidance of obesity which is thought to be closely linked with childhood narcolepsy) and to adopt a positive outlook.

The main *specific* aspect of care is *medication* which is best reserved for children whose lives are significantly affected by their narcolepsy (see Guilleminault & Pelayo (2000) for details including recommended dosage).

Mitler et al. (1994) have reviewed stimulant treatment for narcolepsy in adults, but there have been no properly controlled trials of medication specifically in children. Methylphenidate is often prescribed to combat *sleepiness*, drawing on experience of the use of the drug in the treatment of ADHD. Alternatives have included amphetamines, mazindol and also pemoline which, however, is thought to carry risks of liver damage. The main side-effects of such stimulant drugs are headaches, symptoms of overarousal (such as agitation, tension and anxiety) and gastrointestinal upset. Drug holidays at weekends and during holidays are important to avoid the development of tolerance. Dosage needs to keep pace with physical growth. Modafinil is a recent addition which is unrelated to other CNS stimulant drugs and is said to have fewer adverse psychological effects, including less risk of abuse compared with traditional treatments (McClellan & Spencer, 1998).

Tricyclic drugs, such as clomipramine, have been the main treatment for *cataplexy* (and also for *hallucinations* and *sleep paralysis*). Their main side-effects are dry mouth, constipation and urinary retention. The selective serotonin re-uptake inhibitor fluoxetine is a more recently described alternative.

Unfortunately, *noncompliance* with recommended treatment may be a serious problem, particularly in older children. This can be the result of an unhelpful attitude to the condition, including denial and ambivalence on the part of the child and, sometimes, parents as well.

Additional measures, which may be helpful in their own right without resort to medication in mild cases, include short *planned naps* once or twice a day (mid-afternoon is generally best). This requires careful planning with school to avoid the child being stigmatized as strangely different from other children. Mutual *support groups* are found helpful by some families of affected children.

Other causes of persistent increase in sleep tendency

There appears to be a number of conditions (which may be variations on the theme of narcolepsy or possibly separate conditions) with some but not all of the features of classical narcolepsy. These include narcolepsy without cataplexy but with the characteristic PSG and HLA findings (Parkes et al., 1998).

Other possible causes of excessive daytime sleepiness are as follows:

• The seemingly rare condition of *idiopathic (CNS) hypersomnia* (Billiard, 1996) should be suspected if there is excessive daytime sleepiness, prolonged overnight sleep and great difficulty waking up in the morning or after daytime naps (confusion, disorientation, poor motor co-ordination, slowness and repeated returns to sleep – so called 'sleep drunkenness') but without any of the ancillary clinical symptoms of narcolepsy or PSG features of a REM sleep abnormality. Incomplete forms are described. As the distinction from early narcolepsy may be difficult to make, repeated assessment of the child with these features is necessary. Daytime naps are longer than narcoleptic sleep attacks and also unrefreshing, as already implied.

Age of onset varies from childhood to early adult life. The duration of the disorder seems to be lifelong and its psychological and social effects as serious as narcolepsy. A family pattern of occurrence has been reported, but its genetic basis is unclear and there is no link with HLA antigens. Treatment is similar to that for the sleepiness of narcolepsy.

• Persistent sleepiness may be an aftermath of *infections* such as infectious mono-nucleosis, Lyme disease, Guillain–Barré syndrome and mycoplasma pneu-moniae.

- *Neurological causes* include communicating hydrocephalus, closed head trauma and tumours of the third ventricle or posterior hypothalamus. As mentioned previously, sleepiness may be a feature of many other *chronic medical conditions* such as anaemia or hypothyroidism, or toxic states, although the distinction needs to be made, if possible, between true sleepiness and fatigue or lethargy. The same is true of *depression* and also the *chronic fatigue syndrome* in which various types of sleep disturbance have been reported although often without clear delineation of the underlying sleep disorders (Stores, 1999b). *Medications* which can cause true excessive daytime sleepiness include sedative–hypnotic drugs (barbiturates, benzodiazepines, antihistamines and the newer drugs of this type), sedating antidepressant drugs, and neuroleptic drugs (Obermeyer & Benca, 1996).

- The '*congenital long sleeper*' shows a tendency, starting in childhood, to need more sleep than most other people. This tendency, which may be seen in other members of the family, does not lead to complaints unless (in adolescence in particular) the various social pressures lead to a restriction in sleep duration to levels which would be normal for most other individuals. A sleep diary reveals a consistent pattern of long sleep. The diagnosis rests on the demonstration that there are no clinical or PSG features of any other sleep abnormality leading to excessive sleepiness.

Recurrent hypersomnia

There are a few conditions characterized by periods of excessive sleepiness between which the person spontaneously returns to normal.

- The main example of this pattern is the *Kleine–Levin syndrome* (Bassetti & Aldrich, 2000). In its full classic form, this condition seems to be rare, although it has been suggested that a modified form with only intermittent hypersomnia may be less unusual. The syndrome occurs mainly in males, but occasionally in adolescent females (Kesler et al., 2000), usually begins in middle to late puberty, and often follows an infection or some other type of stressful experience or injury. Periods of hypersomnia (up to 20 hours a day), lasting hours or weeks, occur at intervals of weeks to months. Overeating (sometimes causing obesity) and various forms of hypersexual behaviour occur in the awake state in the classic cases, together with various other disturbances including restlessness, mood disorder, features suggestive of a mild organic confusional state and other behaviours of a bizarre nature. Incomplete forms with only excessive sleepiness are also described. At the end of each episode, a short period of depression or elation with sleeplessness may occur before the sleep pattern and behaviour becomes normal.

  No metabolic or endocrine basis has been established for this condition, and no definitive neurological abnormality has been established. PSG changes during the episodes include a shortened REM latency. Spontaneous improvement over several years is usual. Until this occurs, stimulant drugs are appropriate in severe cases, during the sleepy episodes. There are (inconsistent) reports that further attacks can be prevented by means of tricyclic drugs or lithium (Pike & Stores, 1994). Explanation that the condition is not basically psychological in nature is essential.

CASE: A dispute arose between his parents and his paediatricians about the behaviour of a 10-year-old boy with recurrent episodes over the previous 18 months of apparent daytime sleepiness and bizarre behaviour between which he was his usual normal self. The episodes had begun within 2 days of treatment under a general anaesthetic for a fractured wrist. Each episode consisted of staying in bed asleep for up to 14 hours a day. When awake he indulged in various unusual activities, such as chasing a friend with a carving knife, stealing from the greengrocer's, swimming in his underpants, putting an electric whisk in his mouth and using foul language.

The strangeness of these behaviours, their prompt disappearance at the end of each episode, together with a normal standard EEG recording (taken when the child was not sleepy) were interpreted as evidence of a psychological disorder. The sleepiness was not thought to be genuine. The boy's parents, however, disputed this, pointing out that there was no reason at home or at school why their son should be psychologically disturbed and that his strange behaviour was completely out of character. They insisted that he must have a physical condition and attributed it to the anaesthetic. However, the paediatric team (supported by a child psychiatrist) considered the anaesthetic an unlikely explanation, especially in view of the intermittent nature of the problem.

Reassessment included continuous polysomnography over a 48-hour period. This revealed that the boy was genuinely asleep for the reported long periods. The nature of his sleep and his behaviour were considered characteristic of the Kleine–Levin syndrome. Following prophylactic treatment with lithium, no further episodes have occurred for several years.

Comment: Lack of awareness of this condition, and its surprising features, such as the strange behaviour that can occur and possible precipitation by one or other form of stress, easily lead to the mistaken assumption that the child's behaviour must be psychological in origin even in the absence of definite evidence that this is so.

- Hypersomnia may occur periodically in relation to the *menstrual cycle,* appearing near the start of menarche and resolving spontaneously after months or years. Episodes of this apparently rare condition last about 1 week and resolve at the start of the menses. Oral contraceptives are said to be an effective treatment (Billiard et al., 1975).

- An intermittent pattern may also occur in *recurrent depression* including *seasonal affective disorder (SAD)* which can occur in children and adolescents (see chapter 2) and is characterized by various depressive features, fatigue and overeating, as well as excessive sleepiness or other sleep disturbance, during the winter months, and also response to light therapy (Giedd et al., 1998).

• Other conditions to consider are intermittent *drug abuse,* including the withdrawal phase from stimulant abuse in which extended periods of wakefulness are followed by periods of excessive sleepiness and also REM sleep rebound (Obermeyer & Benca, 1996). Rarely, *nonconvulsive status epilepticus* takes the form of abnormal daytime sleepiness (Stores et al., 1995). Prolonged periods of hypersomnolence apparently triggered by localized *seizures* have also been reported (Wszolek et al., 1995).

Idiopathic recurring stupor is an apparently rare condition of unknown aetiology which should not be confused with recurrent hypersomnia. Patients, without any metabolic, toxic or structural brain disorder, have high plasma and CFS levels of an endogenous benzodiazepine-like substance (endozepine-4) and regular episodes of stupor with widespread fast activity in their EEG. Episodes are promptly resolved by treatment with flumazenil, a benzodiazepine antagonist. The condition has mainly been reported in adults, but examples in children are also described (Soriani et al., 1997).

Excessive sleepiness: basic clinical approach to diagnosis

General

1 Is the problem really excessive sleepiness, or fatigue or lethargy for which different explanations are likely? Check for physical illness or chronic fatigue syndrome.

2 Is the complaint of sleepiness genuine or is it simulated?

3 If sleepiness, how severe is it and what are its effects? (Consider behavioural effects including overactivity in young children.)

4 What form of sleepiness (prolonged overnight sleep, daytime sleepiness including sleep attacks)?

5 Is the sleepiness continuous or intermittent (including worse in winter)?

6 Is the child on any sedating medication? Has he any neurological disorder associated with sleepiness?

At any age

1 Is the child getting sufficient sleep for his age (see sleep duration norms at different ages)?

• How many hours does he usually sleep?

• Does he get to sleep very late but have to get up at a certain time?

• Does he wake up by himself or have to be woken?

• Is it particularly difficult to wake him up and does he resist strongly?

2 Does he sleep soundly?
- Is sleep very restless?
- Is it interrupted by frequent wakings or other disturbance?

3 Is the timing of the sleep period satisfactory?
- Are daytime naps taken inappropriately for child's age?
- Is sleep divided into several periods which are irregular in their distribution or timing (irregular sleep–wake schedule)?
- Does the overnight sleep period seem to be shifted, with difficulty getting to sleep and sleeping in late when possible, e.g. weekends or holidays (delayed sleep phase syndrome)?

4 Specific features:
- Jerky legs during sleep (periodic limb movements)?
- Snoring or other noisy breathing during sleep (upper airway obstruction)? If so:
  - Apnoeic episodes?
  - Other evidence of airway obstruction during sleep?
  - Anatomical features predisposing to upper-airway obstruction?
- Discrete episodes of irresistible sleep during the day? Weakness when excited or alarmed? If so, other features of narcolepsy especially hypnagogic hallucinations, sleep paralysis (narcolepsy syndrome)?
- Sleepiness despite apparently satisfactory sleep (idiopathic hypersomnia)?
- Recurrent periods of excessive sleepiness with normality in between? (See various causes for distinctive features.)

Adolescence

Enquire about characteristic features of:
- Erratic sleep–wake schedules
- Delayed sleep phase syndrome
  - persistently severe difficulty getting to sleep
  - uninterrupted sleep
  - considerable difficulty getting up
  - sleepiness and underfunctioning during the day
  - sleeping in very late at weekends or holidays.
- Other important considerations:
  - tobacco use, caffeine intake?
  - drugs, alcohol abuse?
  - physical illness disrupting sleep?
  - anxiety or depression?
  - other sleep disorder interfering with sleep?
  - motivated to preserve abnormal sleep pattern (school or family problems)?

6

The parasomnias

General aspects

Overnight sleep is not necessarily the quiescent state commonly supposed. There are many physiological processes and behaviours which are initiated or accentuated in relation to sleep and these occur in many people of all ages. Unfortunately, when medical advice is sought for such events, considerable confusion seems to exist about their precise diagnosis and about their psychological or physical significance. These diagnostic uncertainties are often the result of insufficiently detailed descriptions and a general lack of awareness of the many different types of nocturnal disturbance. Uncertainty about the possible significance of the episodes is largely the result of inadequate research.

Definitions and classification

In the ICSD, parasomnias are defined as episodic disorders of arousal, partial arousal, or sleep-stage transition, involving activation of the central nervous system, which intrude into sleep. They are divided into the following four groups according to the stage of sleep with which they are usually associated:

- arousal disorders (usually arising from deep NREM sleep);
- episodes which occur in the transition between wakefulness and sleep;
- parasomnias usually associated with REM sleep;
- other parasomnias which do not fall into these categories and can be associated with various sleep stages.

Parasomnias are classified separately from the dyssomnias (disorders involving difficulty initiating or maintaining sleep, or of excessive sleepiness) and also from mental, neurological or other medical conditions in which sleep disturbance or excessive sleepiness is a major feature.

For general clinical purposes there is merit in considering the parasomnias somewhat differently to this scheme, if only because differential diagnosis frequently crosses the boundaries between parasomnias as defined above and

Table 12. The parasomnias

Primary	Secondary
Sleep onset	*Nocturnal epilepsies*
Sleep starts	
Hypnagogic hallucinations	*Other physical disorders*
Sleep paralysis	Headaches
Rhythmic movement disorder	Respiratory disorders
Restless legs syndrome	Gastrointestinal conditions
	Nocturnal muscle cramps
Light NREM sleep	Cardiac arrhythmias
Bruxism	Sustained sleep starts
Periodic limb movements in sleep	Some cases of restless legs syndrome or
	periodic limb movements in sleep
Deep NREM sleep	
Arousal disorders (confusional arousals,	*Psychiatric disorders*
sleepwalking, sleep terrors)	Post-traumatic stress disorder
	Nocturnal panic attacks
REM sleep	Other (including psychogenic dissociative
Nightmares	states and 'pseudoparasomnias')
REM sleep behaviour disorder	
Waking	
Hypnopompic hallucinations	
Sleep paralysis	
Inconsistently related to stage of sleep	
Sleep talking	
Nocturnal enuresis	
Other primary parasomnias	
Overlap parasomnia disorder	
Sleep-related eating disorder	

psychiatric and medical conditions. From this point of view, parasomnias can be defined as recurrent episodes of behaviour, experiences or physiological changes that occur exclusively or predominantly during or in relation to sleep. Some are *primary* sleep phenomena; others can be considered *secondary* sleep phenomena in that they are manifestations of physical or psychiatric disorder. The primary parasomnias can be subdivided, as just described, according to the stage of sleep or wakefulness in which they typically occur. The main parasomnias classified in this way are shown in Table 12.

Assessment

In general, the main requirement for accurate diagnosis of the parasomnias is careful *clinical assessment* (including the detailed sleep history and other reviews described in chapter 3). *Timing* of the occurrence of the parasomnia has some diagnostic value. This is obviously so for parasomnias occurring at sleep onset or on waking, but it is also important to know that deep NREM sleep (from which arousal disorders usually arise) is largely confined to the first third of the night, and that REM sleep to which certain parasomnias are related is most abundant in the last third. Table 12 shows the typical occurrence of primary parasomnias to illustrate the importance of timing. However, it is particularly important to obtain, as far as possible, all the *subjective and objective details of the onset of the episode and precise sequence of events until the episode is concluded.* The *circumstances of the episodes* should also be described. It should be remembered that a child may have more than one type of parasomnia.

Especially when parents have been alarmed by witnessing the child's night-time episodes, they may be unable to provide sufficient detail, or their account may be distorted with an understandable emphasis on the more dramatic features. In these circumstances, a *diary record* completed at the time, or the use of home *video* (preferably with sound) may provide helpful diagnostic information. Sometimes the audio-video recording conveys a very different picture of the parasomnia from the account given by parents retrospectively in the clinic.

If the diagnosis remains unclear, some form of home-based or inpatient *physiological monitoring* will be required. This can consist of an audio-visual recording with either EEG alone (particularly if epilepsy is suspected), or PSG including respiratory measures, additional EEG channels or anterior tibialis activity monitoring, depending on the type of parasomnia suspected. Other possible uses of PSG in relation to the parasomnias are as follows:

- if the parasomnias are unusual in their nature (including violent or disruptive behaviour), frequency or age of occurrence, or if they persist in spite of seemingly appropriate treatment;
- if there appears to be more than one type of parasomnia;
- where a parasomnia and other forms of sleep disorder may coexist;
- in the diagnosis of REM sleep behaviour disorder with its characteristic preservation of muscle tone in REM sleep;
- to determine whether headbanging or other rhythmic movement disorder is occurring when the child is awake or asleep, in order to choose the most appropriate form of treatment;
- to establish whether the patient is simulating sleep at the time the episodes occur.

Significance

The child's behaviour in many of the parasomnias can be very alarming and parents may well think there must be some serious underlying disorder. As this seems to rarely be the case in children, it is appropriate to reassure the parents that the episodes are very likely to stop of their own accord eventually, although practical measures may be needed, and sometimes treatment, in the meantime.

The challenge is to identify those parasomnias which are not 'developmental' in this sense and which call for attention to the underlying cause. By definition, this will clearly be the case in the secondary parasomnias when they are recognized as such. Research on this point is lacking, but features of primary parasomnias which might indicate that they are symptomatic of a psychological problem are:

- very frequent;
- onset later in development than usual;
- recurrence after having previously stopped;
- persistence into adult life;
- appearance following trauma, suggesting that the parasomnia is one aspect of a post-trauma disorder. The nature of the trauma may be obvious, but, as mentioned previously, sometimes it is covert as in cases of child sexual abuse. Such an experience may be suggested by the content of nightmares or accompanying fears associated with the bedroom setting.

Primary parasomnias related to typical phase of sleep

Presleep and sleep onset

A number of phenomena occur in the process of falling asleep. Most are common in the general population and do not have any pathological significance, despite sometimes causing concern. Sudden, usually single jerks of the limbs or whole body at sleep onset ('*hypnic jerks*') occur at all ages and can be considered normal. In adults, much less-often reported sensory equivalents to these movements include intense flashes of light, a loud bang, crack or snapping noise for which the term 'exploding head syndrome' has been coined (Sachs & Svanborg, 1991), and sudden pain or other unpleasant sensation. Not surprisingly, considerable reassurance may be required that all these so called *sleep starts* are essentially benign, although some association with stress is possible. Their basic nature and frequency of occurrence at any age are not known, but they can be considered a possibility in young patients. Frequent sleep starts have been described in brain-damaged children in whom they may well be interpreted as epileptic in nature (Fusco et al., 1999).

Hypnagogic hallucinations may accompany sleep starts, but often occur separately. As mentioned earlier, they can form part of the narcolepsy syndrome where they can be particularly intense and terrifying. However, the far more usual and isolated form can also be frightening, consisting of a combination of a dreamlike state and awareness of the environment in which objects (including people or animals) may be seen, heard, felt, smelled, tasted or distorted. Body-image distortions may also occur. Again, these experiences, and their counterparts on waking (*hypnopompic hallucinations*), do not usually signify physical or psychological disorder.

Sleep paralysis (Lindsley, 1992) consists of recurrent brief episodes of inability to move or speak, either when going to sleep or on waking, usually from a dream. Eye and respiratory movements are retained, but there is often a feeling of not being able to breathe. The episodes end spontaneously after several seconds to a minute or two, or with external stimulation such as being touched or moved. Sleep paralysis also forms part of the narcolepsy syndrome, but much more often it occurs independently and in rare cases it is familial. As an isolated phenomenon it appears to be common in adults and may well occur in children, although how often is not known. Understandably, it can be very frightening.

The episode of paralysis may be accompanied by hallucinatory experiences or dreamlike experiences which can be very dramatic and alarming, sometimes including the appearance of people or creatures taking on a threatening aspect. Such complaints can be misinterpreted as evidence of psychiatric disorder, including psychotic states (Stores, 1998).

CASE: A 20-year-old with a bipolar affective disorder, began to describe disturbing episodes when he was falling asleep which he had experienced for some years but which he had concealed. Typically, when drifting off to sleep he felt unable to move and saw a small child at the head of his bed who talked with him. More recently, the appearance of this child had become associated with a 'threatening atmosphere' in the bedroom. Sometimes the child seemed to be irritated by the conversations and would sit on the patient's pillow peering at him in a menacing way. At such times the patient felt he could not breathe and became extremely alarmed. Each episode lasted several minutes at most and resolved spontaneously, leaving him frightened for some time afterwards and unable to settle to sleep. These experiences had become increasingly frequent until they were occurring every night.

On enquiry, it seemed that in the past they had been less frequent when the patient was taking tricyclic antidepressant medication. There were no features to suggest the narcolepsy syndrome. As far as could be established, there was no family history of similar experiences.

A diagnosis of isolated (or idiopathic) sleep paralysis with dramatic dream-like accompaniments was made rather than a form of schizophrenia that his psychiatrist had considered based on the apparent hallucinations and delusions including passivity feelings. Treatment with tricyclic medication was recommended in view of its reported beneficial effect on sleep paralysis. However, the patient then read an article in the popular press which said that sleep paralysis might be caused by visitations from extra-terrestrial beings. This intrigued him greatly and he changed from being worried about the night-time events to viewing them as an interesting experience for which he was disinclined to be treated. He eventually moved to another part of the country and was lost to follow up.

Comment: Clearly, to prevent misdiagnosis of this common condition, there is a need for psychiatrists in particular to be well aware of sleep paralysis and the complicated psychological phenomena that can accompany it.

The term *rhythmic movement disorder* (*RMD*) (Thorpy, 1990a) refers to a group of stereotyped movements, mainly of the upper part of the body, usually occurring at sleep onset but also in relation to nocturnal wakings, and sometimes at the end of the sleep period. The reason for such activity has been much debated. In normal children, the activity is pleasurable and may be viewed as at least partly an aid to getting to sleep or returning to sleep following waking during the night. Other examples during NREM or REM sleep have been reported. *Headbanging* is the best-known form, with either forward and backward movement onto a pillow, or perhaps a hard surface such as the cot sides or the wall. Head rolling and rolling or rocking movements of the whole body are in the same category. Combinations of these various movements can occur. Often there are accompanying rhythmic vocalizations such as humming. Individual episodes usually last up to 15 minutes but can be much longer. Many children exhibit some form of sleep-related rhythmic movements in their first year of life, but almost always the behaviour stops spontaneously by 3 to 4 years of age.

In spite of the bizarre nature of RMD in the eyes of parents, it is usually appropriate to reassure them that the behaviour is a passing phase which is not associated with any psychological disorder. Therefore, treatment is not needed except perhaps for protective measures such as padding of the cot sides. In this respect, sleep-related RMD contrasts with that occurring repeatedly during the day, which is often a feature of severe developmental delay or some other form of serious psychiatric condition. Here the risk of head injury from headbanging, including skull trauma and damage to the eyes, appears to be much greater than in sleep-related headbanging.

Occasionally, intervention is necessary because of serious disruption of the child's sleep, embarrassment, annoyance caused to others by the noise generated, or risk of injury. A number of treatments have been reported to be effective in some cases. The various means (described earlier) of helping the child to get to sleep are important, including preventing him spending long periods in bed awake at bedtime. Otherwise, specific behavioural methods, such as the use of reward systems or measures to discourage the movement, may be useful (Golding, 1998). Other psychological treatments said to have been effective (mainly in individual case reports) include measures based on feedback, practising head movements incompatible with actual headbanging, and various reward systems (Owens et al.,

1999a). Occasionally, short-term benzodiazepine medication is justified. Underlying predisposing factors may need attention as in the following case.

CASE: A 4-year-old otherwise normal boy had been banging his head repeatedly every night from the age of 18 months. His parents were distressed by the disruption caused to the whole family, including the patient's brother. Initially the movement consisted of backward banging of his head against the cot rails, but later he converted to banging his head forwards against the side rail of his bed while in a kneeling position. This caused a soft-tissue swelling on his forehead which was noticed by neighbours who reported it to the Social Services department as possible evidence that the boy was being physically abused. Various tranquillizing and sedative medications had been ineffective.

The boy was admitted for investigation, including combined audio-video recording and overnight PSG which demonstrated that he was awake whenever the rhythmic movements took place. The psychologist considered that the movements were being reinforced by the fact that they were eventually followed by sleep each time and substituted a mild negative consequence: each time the movement started he was stood on his feet and briefly walked around the bedroom which he did not like. In addition, not banging his head was rewarded by means of a star chart.

Within 2 weeks the headbanging ceased. It recurred temporarily 6 months later in relation to a family crisis but remitted when the family were able to reinstate the behavioural programme again, and several years later there has been no recurrence.
Comment: the case illustrates the effectiveness of behavioural treatment over medication, and also how family factors influence the implementation of treatment.

Restless legs syndrome (discussed earlier) can be viewed as a form of parasomnia causing difficulty getting to sleep.

Light sleep (NREM stages 1 and 2)

Bruxism or *teethgrinding* (Bader & Lavigne, 2000) is forcible grinding and clenching of the teeth in a paroxysmal fashion, producing a loud grinding noise at night without the child being aware. This usually occurs in light sleep, but may occur at any stage of sleep. It is thought to be very common and to be caused by a number of physical or psychological factors, although its origin may not be clear. Stress may precipitate or exacerbate the condition. The child may complain of pain in the face or headache. In severe cases, the child's teeth might be damaged. Treatment, if needed, is determined by the cause or associated factors, but the range of suggested remedies in adults (from orthodontic manœuvres to psychotherapy and even hypnotherapy) indicates the need for careful consideration of each individual case and for further research on this topic.

Periodic limb movements in sleep were also discussed earlier in the section on excessive sleepiness. Although classified in the ICSD as an intrinsic cause of insomnia, this condition can also be grouped here under the broad definition of the parasomnias.

Deep sleep (NREM stages 3 and 4): arousal disorders (Thorpy, 1990b)
General points

The so-called disorders of arousal (i.e. confusional arousals, sleepwalking and sleep terrors) are very common parasomnias in childhood. Arousal in this context does not mean that the child wakes up; the arousal is, in fact, a *partial arousal* usually from deep NREM sleep (SWS) to another lighter stage of NREM sleep or REM sleep. In such arousals, a range of behaviours can occur. These can be simple, for example sitting up in bed and mumbling, or complicated, such as rushing out of the house in a highly agitated state. The child remains asleep during the episode itself, although waking sometimes occurs immediately afterwards.

Typically, there is only one episode on the night in question, within the first 2 hours or so after going to sleep when SWS is most abundant. However, some children predisposed to arousal disorders also have such arousals arising from light NREM and REM sleep, giving rise to multiple episodes throughout the night (Naylor & Aldrich, 1991). Such repeated episodes are usually less dramatic each time. Although young children may have a further period of SWS at the end of the sleep period, it is unusual for such partial arousals to occur towards getting up time. Partial arousals are possible during daytime naps.

Rosen et al. (1995) list the following *constitutional or predisposing factors*:
- genetic (a parental history of partial arousals has been reported in up to 60% of cases);
- young age (when SWS is very deep and long lasting);
- sleep loss or disruption, or irregular sleep–wake patterns (making full arousal from SWS difficult);
- the sleep-disruptive effects of stress or trauma.

Other, ill-defined associations include that between sleepwalking and migraine (Barabas et al., 1983).

Precipitating factors include:
- fever;
- systemic illness;
- CNS depressant medication;
- internal or external sleep-interrupting stimuli (including the child being woken forcefully);
- other sleep disorders in which sleep is interrupted, such as OSA;
- psychological factors which may precipitate or maintain the occurrence of the episodes and also influence their severity.

Significance

Arousal disorders are important in a number of ways.

- They often worry parents who think the more dramatic forms mean the child is psychologically disturbed. Professionals (including psychiatrists) may share this concern which, in fact, seems rarely justified, unlike (it has been claimed) the occurrence of arousal disorder in adults (Ohayon et al., 1999) and also in adolescents (Gau & Soong, 1999). However, referral bias in these reported series of patients is a possibility.
- They can be embarrassing for children themselves, especially if they occur away from home.
- They are often confused with other primary or secondary parasomnias.
- They carry a risk of accidental injury.
- Rarely, the child's behaviour may endanger others causing serious injury (Oswald & Evans, 1985), although less so than in adults.
- Occasionally, they indicate underlying psychological disturbance. The possible pointers to this were mentioned earlier.

Types of arousal disorder

Three main forms of arousal disorder are described, although episodes may combine elements of all three. Sleepwalking and sleep terrors are well known; confusional arousals are generally less well recognized. Clinically, all have in common a curious combination of features suggestive of being simultaneously awake and asleep. Despite seeming to be alert (indeed sometimes highly aroused) depending on the type of arousal disorder, the following general factors are apparent:

- confusion and disorientation;
- remaining asleep during the episode, although in later childhood and subsequently (unlike earlier) there is a tendency to wake up at the end of an episode;
- unresponsiveness to environmental events including parents' attempts to communicate with the child;
- little or (usually) no recall of events during each episode of disturbed behaviour.

The child might display a sequence of confusional arousals in early childhood, sleepwalking later, then sleep terrors in late childhood and adolescence. Alternatively, elements of all three forms can occur at any one stage of development. Similarly, the family history of arousal disorder can take a variety of forms.

Confusional arousals occur mainly in infants and toddlers perhaps most of whom have such episodes to some degree. An episode may begin with movements and moaning and then progress to agitated and confused behaviour with crying (perhaps intense), calling out, or thrashing about. Typically, although appearing alert, the child does not respond when spoken to, but more forceful attempts to intervene may meet with resistance and increased agitation.

Parents are often very alarmed and, wanting to console the child, they may make vigorous attempts to waken him, without success or only with much trying. Such efforts may actually prolong the arousal and, if the child is woken to some extent, he is likely to be confused and frightened. Each episode usually lasts 5–15 minutes (possibly much longer) before the child calms down spontaneously and returns to restful sleep.

Sleepwalking is said to occur in up to 17% of children (usually sporadically) mainly between 4 and 8 years of age. Episodes, which can last up to 10 minutes or so, are usually less dramatic than confusional arousals. The young child may crawl or walk about in his cot. At a later age, he may calmly walk around his room or into other parts of the house such as to the toilet, towards a light or to his parents' bedroom. The child may appear downstairs or may be found standing on the landing or elsewhere in the house, looking vague with eyes open but with a glassy stare. At most, he will be partially responsive. Some children are found asleep in various parts of the house. Quite complicated routes may be followed if well known to the child, or other complex habitual behaviour (automatism) may occur possibly extending over long periods of time. Urinating in inappropriate places is common.

Accidental injury in sleepwalking (e.g. from falling downstairs) is a serious risk. In later childhood or adolescence, the wandering may extend further within the house or outside. At this age and later, the sleepwalking may take an *agitated form* which also may be worsened by attempts to intervene and with an even greater risk of injury from crashing through windows or glass doors, for example.

CASE: A 5-year-old girl was the subject of a possible child protection order because the Social Services department suspected that she had been thrown out of her bedroom window by her father about whom there were other suspicions concerning his conduct within the family. The girl was found late one evening lying on the patio pavement under her first-floor bedroom window which was open. She had fallen face down and broken both her wrists. Her parents insisted that the window was routinely fastened closed. To have opened it, the girl had to have climbed on to a chest of drawers, slid the inner double-glazing panel sideways, and unfastened the window catch before swinging the window open and climbing through.

The social work team considered that this sequence of actions was too complicated to have been performed in the course of sleepwalking. The child's parents insisted this must have happened in view of her other frequent sleepwalking episodes during the previous 2 years. There was a strong family history on mother's side of sleepwalking and night terrors.

Following explanation that complicated habitual behaviour is possible in sleepwalking episodes, the intention to take the child into care was abandoned. A programme of treatment for the sleepwalking was instituted consisting of scheduled waking (see later). Further attempts to improve relationships between the family members were also made.

Comment: It is often not appreciated (including in the legal context) that complicated behaviour is possible during a sleepwalking episode. However, there needs to be convincing evidence that the person suffers from an arousal disorder and that the actions during the episode are of a type that is compatible with this interpretation of the behaviour (Broughton et al., 1994).

Night terrors ('pavor nocturnus') are better called *sleep terrors* as they are associated with sleep, whenever its timing. They occur in about 3% of children mainly in later childhood. The natural history of this and other arousal disorders have been little studied. Preliminary reports suggest that sleep terrors starting before about 7 years of age continue on average for about 4 years, and that those of later onset tend to last much longer (Dimario & Emery, 1987).

Classically, parents are woken by their child's piercing scream which marks the very sudden onset of the partial arousal. The child appears to be terrified, with staring eyes, intense sweating, rapid pulse and cries or other vocalizations suggesting intense distress. He may jump out of bed and rush about frantically, as if trying to escape from something. Injury from running into furniture or jumping through windows is again a serious risk. Other people may also be injured in the process. The event usually lasts no more than a few minutes at most. Typically it ends abruptly and the child settles back to sleep. If he wakes up at the end of the episode, the child may describe a feeling of primitive threat or danger, but not the extended narrative of a nightmare.

Differential diagnosis

If a detailed clinical description is obtained, special investigations are not usually necessary for the recognition of arousal disorders. However, PSG might be helpful if, despite careful clinical evaluation, the distinction still cannot be made between arousals and the other parasomnias (described later) which can involve complicated behaviour at night. That is not to say that the PSG between episodes should be expected to contain features specifically diagnostic of arousal disorders. However, there is some evidence that people with this type of sleep disorder can have unusually high levels of SWS but difficulty sustaining it. This difficulty is suggested by frequent shifts from SWS to another level of sleep, abnormal amounts of hypersynchronous slow (delta) EEG activity and rapidly induced arousals, together with frequent brief microarousals (Blatt et al., 1991). A combination of clinical and PSG findings (preferably obtained during the episodes in question) may help to distinguish arousal disorders and the following episodic events described in this and other chapters:

- true nightmares (as distinct from the loose use of the term 'nightmare' for any dramatic behavioural disturbance at night);
- some types of nocturnal epileptic seizures;
- 'awakenings' associated with OSA;
- gastro-oesophageal reflux;
- REM sleep behaviour disorder;
- nocturnal panic attacks which, however, have been described in combination with arousal disorders (Garland & Smith, 1991);
- episodes at night which appear to be parasomnias but which are shown by PSG to be enacted when the child is actually awake (Molaie & Deutch, 1997).

Perhaps the most usual *diagnostic confusions* concern the differences between partial arousals, nightmares and nocturnal seizures. Their main features are shown in Table 13.

Treatment of arousal disorders

- Parents' anxiety is usually lessened by *explanation with reassurance* (where justified) that these often dramatic and frightening events do not mean that the child is ill or disordered, and that he can be expected to grow out of them.
- General principles of *regular and adequate sleep routines* (to prevent loss or disruption of sleep) are important.
- Parents should be encouraged to *make the environment as safe as possible* to reduce the risk of injury, for example remove obstructions in the bedroom, secure windows, locks or alarms on outside doors or cover windows with heavy curtains.
- They should be encouraged to *refrain from trying to waken or restrain the child* during the episode. As mentioned, waking the child is difficult, counterproductive (the child will be confused and frightened if wakened forcefully) and unnecessary. It is much better to wait until the episode subsides and calmly help the child back to quiet sleep.
- If the child has no recall of the episodes, there is *little point in recounting them*, as this may become a source of anxiety.
- If sleepwalking or sleep-terror episodes are frequent and consistent in their time of occurrence, '*scheduled awakening*' can be helpful (Frank et al., 1997). This consists of the child being gently and briefly woken 15–30 minutes before the episode is due. This procedure is repeated nightly for up to a month. Preliminary reports suggest that improvement can be maintained for at least several months. Concern has been expressed that sometimes this form of treatment causes such loss of sleep that the arousal disorder becomes more severe (Owens et al., 1999a).
- *Medication* should be reserved for particularly worrying, embarrassing or dangerous arousals where other measures have failed. Benzodiazepines (such as

Table 13. Comparison of main features of partial arousals, nightmares and nocturnal seizures

	Partial arousals	Nightmares	Nocturnal seizures[a]
Time of the night	Usually first third of the night	Middle to last third of the night	Variable
Usual stage of sleep	Deep NREM	REM	Variable
Behaviour	Variable but usually dramatic apart from calm sleepwalking; often inaccessible and cannot be comforted; may resist intervention	Distressed by frightening dream, accessible and welcomes comforting	Variable, may be undirected violence or distress during or after attack
Level of consciousness	Unaware during episode, confused if awakened or following episode	Asleep during episode, fully awake afterwards	Variable
Likelihood of injury	Moderate	Low	Low
Memory for events	None	Vivid recall	Variable
Family history	Common	None	Variable
Prevalence	Common	Common	Much less common

[a]In view of the wide range of types of epileptic seizure associated with sleep, the descriptions given are generalizations with certain clear exceptions to the general rule (see text).

low-dose clonazepam) and tricyclic drugs (e.g. imipramine) have been used but with mixed results. There is some evidence that selective serotonin reuptake inhibitors might be effective (Lillywhite et al., 1994). Use of benzodiazepines is best restricted to several weeks at most to avoid possible hazards of long-term use (e.g. tolerance, adverse effects and abuse) although reassuring findings about such risks have been reported in adults where extended use has seemed justified because of the serious nature of their arousal disorders or other parasomnia (Schenck & Mahowald, 1996). Underlying mechanisms of action are unclear, but it is thought the effect of medication is less the result of reduction of SWS associated with these drugs than their influence on the arousal response.

- If there is evidence of an *underlying psychological problem*, appropriate enquiries and help will be needed.

REM sleep parasomnias

Being frightening dreams, *nightmares* are the obvious example of a REM sleep-related parasomnia (Maurer & Schaefer, 1998). However, caution is needed with the term 'nightmare' because, as already mentioned, it is sometimes used mistakenly for any type of recurrent dramatic night-time episode. On occasions, 'nightmare' and 'night terror' are used interchangeably, or one is thought to be a variety of the other. Nightmares are sometimes called 'dream anxiety attacks'.

True nightmares, which typically occur in the later part of overnight sleep when REM sleep is most abundant, are very common from early childhood (up to about 50% of children overall), although their content varies with age, tending to become increasingly complex. Typically, the child wakes up, very frightened and fully alert, and relates his fear to a vividly recalled sequence of dream events, often involving the child himself or someone well known. The child remains afraid after waking up and cannot get back to sleep for some time, although it is usually possible to reassure and comfort him.

Generally, such dreams occur infrequently without any serious psychological significance. They may be spontaneous or (like partial arousals) precipitated by illness and psychological stress of any sort. As discussed shortly, they are a prominent part of PTSD and their content may be revealing, especially if consistent. In such circumstances, nightmares may well coexist with bedtime fears. The many medications whose use is associated with their occurrence include antidepressants and neuroleptics. Abrupt withdrawal from REM-suppressing substances (including most antidepressants, benzodiazepines, methylphenidate and alcohol) can precipitate nightmares because of a REM sleep rebound effect later in the night.

Occasional nightmares require no special measures apart from comforting the child at the time they occur. Preventive measures include avoidance of disturbing stories or videos before going to bed. Owens et al (1999a) point to the very limited research on psychological forms of treatment for nightmares. Measures which are thought might be helpful include systematically helping the child to be less concerned about the frightening content of the nightmare, or rehearsing the content but with a modified, less alarming ending. In more complicated cases, treatment is that of the underlying cause including the use of various forms of psychotherapy.

REM sleep behaviour disorder (Mahowald & Schenck, 2000) is a relatively newly described parasomnia. It was initially thought to be confined to elderly men, but recent reports indicate that it (or a similar disorder) can occur in other groups including children (Sheldon & Jacobsen, 1998). It is characterized by pathological preservation of muscle tone during REM sleep which allows dreams to be acted out. If the dreams are violent, the patient punches, kicks, leaps or runs about, often causing self-injury or injury to anyone nearby.

In adults, the classic form is often associated with neurodegenerative disease (especially Parkinson's disease) and narcolepsy. It has also been reported in association with juvenile Parkinson's disease (Rye et al., 1999). It is thought that the remaining idiopathic variety may often be the early sign of a neuro-degenerative disorder (Montagna, 2000) and that lesser forms of REM sleep motor dysfunction (especially with sleeptalking) can be an even earlier sign (Tachibana et al., 1997). A major stress seems to have triggered the onset of the condition in some cases. Because of these strong associations with organic factors, REM sleep behaviour disorder can actually be considered a secondary parasomnia in many cases. An *acute form* has been described in adults associated with the use or withdrawal of alcohol, various antidepressant drugs, amphetamines and clonidine.

Diagnosis rests on a combination of sleep-related injury or disruptive behaviour with evidence from audio-visual/PSG monitoring of increased muscle tone or phasic twitching in REM sleep, prominent movements or vigorous jerking often with intense vocalizations in REM sleep, and recall of corresponding dream content on waking. Clonazepam is an effective treatment in most cases.

Obviously, REM sleep behaviour disorder is of clinical and forensic importance as a possible cause of *sleep-related violence.* Other possible explanations for such behaviour include arousal disorder, organic confusional states at night, nocturnal epilepsy (rarely), OSA awakenings and psychologically determined states (Broughton & Shimizu, 1997). Although there are few reports of REM sleep behaviour disorder in children, it should be considered as a possible explanation of dramatic nocturnal behaviour.

CASE: A 29-year-old man was referred to the sleep disorders clinic because he frequently acted out his dreams at night. He had been doing this since the age of 14, but concern about his behaviour had increased within the last 2 years because of injuries inflicted on his partner and because their 5-month-old daughter had to share her parents' bedroom because of the family's limited living accommodation.

The patient reported that in his early teens he had acted out pleasurably exciting dreams, but later he began to enact different dreams, including those with a violent content in the course of which he had damaged bedroom furniture. More recently, he had injured his partner when dreaming, for example, that she was being attacked during the night by someone from whom he had to wrestle her free. On other occasions he had injured himself and damaged the bedroom door when acting out a dream that he was repelling people coming up the stairs to attack him and his family.

The frequency of these episodes had increased to 4–5 times a week. They usually occurred in the later part of the night, up to 5 a.m. He was described as a restless sleeper with much moaning and groaning. He reported feeling tired during the day. He exhibited no other abnormal features either when awake or asleep.

The patient had a past history of family and school problems followed by a period of excessive alcohol intake, use of illicit substances and aggression. However, in recent times his general behaviour and conduct had been unremarkable. There was no relationship between his dreams and taking medication. The family history included alcoholism and violence but no known neurological disease or severe sleep disorder.

At the time of referral, no abnormality was found on physical examination and his mental state and intellectual level were judged to be normal. Investigations included brain MRI which was normal. Extended PSG produced evidence of both REM sleep behaviour disorder and also frequent periodic limb movements in sleep often associated with arousals. There were no findings to suggest any other form of sleep disorder. Clonazepam was prescribed, and soon after the violent dreams and behaviour stopped and the patient's sleep became generally more restful.

Comment: An intriguing aspect of this case is the early age of onset of the REM sleep behaviour disorder. This was unrelated to psychotropic or any other medication, alcohol excess or drug misuse, and without any evidence at the time, or in the following 15 years, of narcolepsy or other underlying neurological disorder. The patient remains under review for any further developments that might explain the origin of his condition.

Waking

The two main parasomnias occurring at the time of waking are *hypnopompic hallucinations* and *sleep paralysis*, both of which were described earlier as examples of parasomnias at the onset of sleep.

Primary parasomnias inconsistently related to stages of sleep

Sleeptalking is common and occurs in all sleep stages. It occurs as an isolated phenomenon but can also be a feature of a variety of other sleep disorders, such as arousal disorders, OSA or REM sleep behaviour disorder. Sleeptalking is usually spontaneous but may be in response to conversation. It is usually brief and inconsequential but sometimes it extends to long speeches, possibly emotional in tone. At times it consists only of moaning noises. By itself, sleeptalking is of no clinical significance apart from the annoyance caused to others trying to sleep nearby. Treatment is difficult to specify unless there is a particular underlying sleep disorder.

Nocturnal enuresis (*bedwetting*) is a particularly common problem in children (Challamel & Cochat, 1999). A diagnosis of nocturnal enuresis implies recurrent involuntary bedwetting in the absence of an organic cause in a child over the age of 5 years. A commonly used mnemonic is that 10% of 5 year olds and 5% of 10 year olds wet the bed. However, published prevalence rates vary according to the frequency of bedwetting reported, and from one country to another. Bedwetting at least once a week occurs in about 5% of 7 year olds and 3% of 9 year olds. Around 2% are still affected at age 11 years and perhaps 1% at age 14 years or older. No apparent decrease has occurred in the last 40 years or more (Rona et al., 1997). Boys outnumber girls increasingly as childhood advances. Children are said to have *primary enuresis* if they have never achieved normal bladder control (accounting for 70–90% of cases); *secondary enuresis* means loss of control after acquiring it for at least 6 months.

Various possible *causes or associated factors* have been described:
- enuresis can be seen as a *maturational problem* which is often shared by other family members;
- *limited functional bladder capacity* or *bladder instability*;
- *parental failure to toilet train the child satisfactorily*;
- *overall developmental delay*;
- *behavioural disturbance*;
- *social disadvantage*;
- *stressful experiences* of any type (psychological factors seem to be more relevant in the development of secondary enuresis).

Nocturnal enuresis can be a cause of embarrassment and upset for the child (restricting social activities away from home), and annoyance and even punitive behaviour on the part of parents.

Although once considered to be an arousal disorder and still often regarded as a result of particularly deep sleep, enuresis can occur in any stage of sleep. As it may be associated with OSA and (unusually) with partial arousals, a complete sleep history should be taken. By means of careful history taking, physical examination and urinalysis, enuresis should be distinguished from organic causes of bedwetting including urinary tract infection (especially girls), structural abnormalities of the urinary tract, diabetes insipidus and neurological conditions (including epilepsy) in which bedwetting (and possibly also wetting by day) are liable to occur.

A number of *treatment approaches* have been described (Moffatt, 1997) such as the following.
- Basic measures such as *fluid restriction* before bedtime or *waking* the child to go to the toilet before the parents go to bed have often been recommended, but these practices may be of little help.
- *Behavioural approaches* include *rewards* for dry nights rather than recriminations when the child wets the bed. *Conditioning* by means of an alarm system is reported to be effective in a high proportion of cases if attempted in a systematic, consistent and determined way, including overlearning beyond the initial positive response. The relapse rate is said to be relatively low.

- *Medication* in the form of desmopressin (DDAVP) and low-dose tricyclic antidepressants (e.g. imipramine) are said to be effective second-line treatments but with a high relapse rate when withdrawn. Because of the potential cardiotoxic effects of the tricyclic drugs, desmopressin is often preferred for short-term use or for special circumstances, e.g. when staying with friends for a brief period.
- *Bladder training* to increase bladder capacity and stability.
- Negative *attitudes* to the child.
- *Psychiatric help* should be provided in the few cases where this is appropriate.

Other primary parasomnias

Some parasomnias appear to combine elements from the different categories just described. Schenck et al. (1997) have reported an '*overlap parasomnia disorder*' in patients of various ages (including children and adolescents) exhibiting clinical and PSG features of sleepwalking, sleep terrors and REM sleep behaviour disorder. Some patients had physical or psychiatric disorders; in others the condition seems to be idiopathic.

Examples described in adults of parasomnias with mixed states of wakefulness and the different sleep stages (Mahowald & Schenk, 1992) mean that traditional diagnostic criteria in characterizing an individual's parasomnia may need to be relaxed. For example, this may be the case in the parasomnias associated with PTSD, as discussed shortly. *Sleep-related eating disorders* (Schenck et al., 1993) illustrate how strange behaviour at night can be a feature of various underlying sleep disorders. Mainly a problem in females, the often bizarre eating practices at night may begin in childhood. The association with daytime eating disorder is debated, some claiming that it is often overlooked in those with a daytime eating problem (Winkelman et al., 1999). The behaviour is mainly linked to sleepwalking but may also occur in people with OSA, restless legs syndrome, narcolepsy, or other causes of disrupted sleep. Treatment is that of the underlying sleep disorder.

It is important to consider that a child may have *more than one type of parasomnia*. This may be either more than one primary parasomnia or a combination of a primary parasomnia and a parasomnia secondary to physical or psychiatric disorder, such as night terrors with nocturnal epilepsy (Tassinari et al., 1972).

Secondary parasomnias

The secondary parasomnias illustrate very well that it is important for clinicians in all specialties to be aware of the sleep-related manifestations of psychiatric and other medical disorders. They are also a reminder that the possibility of an underlying illness must be considered in the case of episodic disturbances at night, although the likelihood of this seems less in children than at other ages.

Nocturnal epilepsies

Possibly the main source of uncertainty about distinguishing between the primary and secondary parasomnias concerns the nocturnal occurrence of epileptic attacks ('seizures'). Sleep disorders can be confused with epilepsy and vice versa (Stores, 1991). These are important mistakes because the significance of epilepsy is very different from most primary parasomnias in terms of underlying cause, the need for special investigations, the type of treatment required and ultimate prognosis.

Few generalizations about 'epilepsy' are justified because the term covers such a wide range of conditions which are different in their cause, manifestations, effects, treatment needs and natural history (Commission on Classification and Terminology of the International League Against Epilepsy, 1989). This diversity is reflected in those epilepsies in which seizures occur at night. The varied clinical manifestations of nocturnal seizures makes it difficult to generalize about the features which distinguish such seizures from other parasomnias (Table 13).

There are a number of types of epilepsy, both generalized and localized, in which the seizures are closely related to the sleep–wake cycle (Autret et al., 1999). In some, the seizures are relatively subtle and may go undetected at night; in others the seizure manifestations are more dramatic, creating a greater risk of diagnostic confusion.

- *Mesial frontal seizures* illustrate this problem well (Stores et al., 1991). This not uncommon form of epilepsy is often misdiagnosed. The main reason is the complicated motor manifestations (e.g. kicking, hitting, rocking, thrashing and cycling or scissor movements of the legs) and vocalizations (from grunting, coughing, muttering or moaning to shouting, screaming or roaring) which characterize these seizures. The abrupt onset and termination, short duration of the attacks (different from seizures of temporal lobe origin) and, sometimes, preservation of consciousness can also suggest a nonepileptic basis for the attacks. Diagnosis rests on awareness of this form of epilepsy and recognition of these clinical features. EEG recordings even during the episodes are of limited diagnostic value. The underlying cerebral pathology varies, and often no structural abnormality is found. One form is clearly genetic in origin with an autosomal dominant pattern (Scheffer et al., 1995). It is considered likely that the brief type of *nocturnal paroxysmal dystonia* is, in fact, this form of epilepsy (Tinuper et al., 1990). Response to treatment seems very variable.

CASE: For the previous 4 years a 12-year-old girl had been having frequent stereotyped night-time attacks, with many of the features just described, which had been diagnosed as 'nightmares' despite there being no evidence of frightening dreams. Similar episodes during the day were said to be 'pseudoseizures' although no psychological reason could be identified.

Reassessment included PSG with additional EEG channels emphasizing frontal electrode placements. The recordings demonstrated a source of seizure discharge in the left frontal area, with localized seizure activity accompanying many of her attacks both by day and by night. Neuroimaging revealed no structural abnormality. Treatment with carbamazepine was introduced. The attacks gradually ceased over the following few months.

Comment: The case illustrates the delay and misdiagnosis which commonly occurs in this form of epilepsy. Response to treatment was good in this patient but is not always the case.

- The manifestation of *seizures of temporal lobe origin* may well have features in common with some of the more dramatic types of primary parasomnias, at least in older children (Brockhaus & Elger, 1995). This includes those seizures with prominent affective symptoms, especially fear.
- Fear is also prominent in *benign epilepsy with affective symptoms* (Dalla Bernardina et al., 1992) in which nocturnal seizures usually appear soon after falling asleep.
- *Benign partial epilepsy with centro-temporal spikes* or *Rolandic epilepsy* (Loiseau & Duché, 1989) is a common form of childhood epilepsy in which about 75% of patients have their seizures exclusively during sleep. The oropharyngeal motor, sensory and autonomic symptoms of this form of epilepsy, often with preservation of consciousness, can be very distressing to the child, giving rise to disturbed behaviour. The seizures occur on falling asleep, in the middle of the night or (perhaps mainly) shortly before or on waking. Diagnosis rests mainly on the clinical characteristics of the episodes, but interictal centro-temporal spikes with normal background EEG activity is an important confirmatory finding.
- In *benign occipital epilepsy* (Gastaut, 1992) the seizures themselves (which may involve complex visual experiences including hallucinations and illusions) and the child's reactions can involve dramatic behaviour. A mainly nocturnal form with early onset (mainly around the age of 5 years) has been described (Panayiotopoulos, 2000).
- *Paroxysmal awakenings, paroxysmal sleeptalking* and *episodic nocturnal wanderings* are other forms of sleep-related conditions with prominent motor manifestations which are now thought to be forms of frontal lobe epilepsy (Provini et al., 1999). These authors suggest that agitated sleepwalking and high-frequency motor events, or those which persist beyond puberty, may well also be frontal seizures.

The distinction between epilepsy and other parasomnias (and indeed between the various types of nocturnal seizures) should be possible in most cases by careful clinical evaluation combined with the appropriate special investigations. As emphasized previously, the main requirement is as detailed an account as possible of the sequence of events from the start of each episode until the child has recovered, together with a description of the circumstances in which the episode occurred. Special investigations include sleep studies and long-term EEG monitoring by various means such as combined video/EEG monitoring, or home EEG monitoring which is generally more acceptable to children (Stores, 1985). The occurrence of attacks both at night and during the day favours epilepsy. However, the diagnosis may remain difficult because of the variable clinical manifestations and EEG accompaniments of some seizures.

CASE: Advice was sought from the sleep clinic about a 10-year-old girl from another part of the country who, 12 months previously, had begun to have episodes of disturbed behaviour during the night sometimes lasting several minutes. Typically, she appeared to be suddenly terrified, with profuse sweating, staring, reddening of the face, before rushing about the bedroom screaming. The first episode usually occurred within about 2 hours of going to sleep, followed by further attacks up to 20 times throughout the night. There was no past personal history of sleep disturbance or other disorder and nothing in the family history of obvious significance.

EEG investigations, including recording through several of her night-time attacks, had revealed no definite abnormality, although one standard inter-attack recording was thought to contain infrequent sharp wave discharges in the right mid-temporal region. A structural MRI scan was reported as normal, and basic tests for neurodegenerative disease had contained no abnormality.

Largely on the basis of the EEG findings, a diagnosis of sleep terrors had been made, but the referring paediatrician had reservations about this. The child's episodes recorded on video were reviewed. It was considered that their abrupt onset and termination, relatively short duration, frequent occurrence, close relationship to sleep and (in particular) the complex automatisms and vocalizations, with a strong affective content, raised the possibility of mesial frontal epilepsy.

Contrary to advice, no further investigations were performed by the referring clinical service, and a therapeutic trial of antiepileptic medication was undertaken. This was promptly followed by a reduction and then cessation of the child's attacks.

Comment: Despite the inconclusive diagnosis, it seems likely that the patient had been suffering a form of epilepsy initially misdiagnosed as night terrors. Symptoms of these two very different disorders can overlap, but the absence of earlier signs of an arousal disorder, the negative family history, and the very high frequency of the episodes, as well as the features suggesting mesial frontal epilepsy make the diagnosis of epilepsy very likely. The largely negative EEG findings (including those obtained during the episodes) are compatible with epilepsy, especially of mesial frontal origin.

Further points concerning distinctions between nocturnal epilepsy and other types of sleep disorder areas follows.

- In adults, *epilepsy has been misdiagnosed as sleep apnoea* where seizures have involved awakenings with feelings of choking, abnormal movements and excessive daytime sleepiness (Oldani et al., 1998).

- *OSA can be a cause of anoxic seizures* (Cirignotta et al., 1989).
- *Seizures of primarily cerebral origin may be exacerbated by a concomitant sleep disorder*, for example seizures have been reported to improve with treatment of sleep apnoea in children (Koh et al., 2000).
- *Periodic limb movements in sleep* are sometimes mistaken for seizures (Picchietti & Walters, 1999).
- *Repetitive sleep starts* described in neurologically impaired children and easily mistaken for myoclonic seizures (Fusco et al., 1999), further illustrate the need for careful diagnosis of paroxysmal events, especially in such children, in this case to avoid overstating the frequency of genuine seizures.
- *Epilepsy during sleep may be simulated* by patients who are actually awake (Thacker et al., 1993).

Other parasomnias of physical origin (Mahowald & Schenck, 1996)

Illustrations were given earlier of organic factors which can precipitate arousal disorders, for instance, in susceptible individuals. In other circumstances, the parasomnia is a manifestation of the physical disorder itself. Examples in children include:

- *headaches* of a migrainous type (sometimes related to REM sleep);
- *respiratory disorders* such as asthma or sleep apnoea (including recognizable types of parasomnia and also awakenings often of an ill-defined nature);
- *gastro-intestinal conditions*, notably gastro-oesophageal reflux and diffuse oesophageal spasm;
- nocturnal *muscle cramps*;
- *cardiac arrhythmias*;
- *restless legs syndrome* and *periodic limb movements in sleep*, both of which can be symptomatic of an underlying physical illness such as a metabolic disorder;
- as described previously, *REM sleep behaviour disorder* may well be secondary to neurological disease or medication.

Parasomnias secondary to psychiatric disorders

Mention has already been made of the part played by stress in triggering various parasomnias in children predisposed to them. However, the concern here is with primary psychiatric disorders, the clinical manifestations of which include episodic disturbances of behaviour or experience and which, therefore, call for psychiatric help rather than attention to the sleep disorder alone.

When the significance of childhood parasomnias was discussed earlier, it was suggested that certain features might alert the clinician to the need to make further enquiries about a possible underlying psychological problem. In the absence of sound information on this point, it was suggested that these features might include the frequency of occurrence of the parasomnia, age at which the episodes began or recurred, and sometimes their content. Onset following trauma strongly suggests a more generalized emotional disorder, although the traumatic experience (notably sexual abuse) may not be obvious and may need sensitive enquiries to elicit its occurrence and nature.

- As mentioned earlier, sleep disturbance is acknowledged to be a prominent feature of *post-traumatic stress disorder* (PTSD). Indeed, it has been suggested that REM sleep disturbance might be the basis for many of the symptoms of the condition, although this notion has been disputed (Reynolds, 1989). Emphasis has been placed mainly on 'nightmares' but, again, in the loose sense of this term to include various dramatic parasomnias in adults, some of which do not seem to fit into conventional categories (Kramer et al., 1984). The limited information available suggests that the sleep disturbance in children with PTSD extends beyond parasomnias, including excessive daytime sleepiness (Sheldon et al., 1991).

  There is a need to study the details of effects of different types of trauma on children of different ages, and to explore the possible benefits of more focussed treatment of the sleep disturbance as part of the overall care of such children. By sleeping better, the child is likely to be more able to cope with the other effects of being traumatized.

CASE: For the previous 5 years, a 7-year-old girl had experienced recurrent episodes throughout nearly every night in which she rhythmically rolled from side to side, for up to 5 minutes each time. Occasionally, she also banged her head backwards on the pillow repeatedly. Some time before referral to the sleep clinic she had been diagnosed as having nocturnal epilepsy, but had not responded to anti-epileptic medication which she was still taking at the time she was referred.

Extended overnight PSG with audio-visual monitoring demonstrated recurrent waking episodes with body rolling, sometimes accompanied by moaning and apparent brief cries of distress, without evidence of epileptic activity of any type. A diagnosis of persistent rhythmic movement disorder was made and the anti-epileptic treatment was withdrawn.

The question arose why her sleep was so often interrupted (the rhythmic movements were interpreted as an aid to getting back to sleep). Careful enquiry revealed that for some years she had been the victim of sexual abuse. The recurrent awakenings were viewed as part of the emotional distress that this had caused. Extensive work with the family was carried out by psychiatric colleagues. The awakenings and rhythmic movements gradually remitted over the next 2 years.

Comment: The case illustrated the risk that epilepsy will be diagnosed too readily without adequate assessment and an appreciation of other types of nocturnal events. It also emphasized the need to consider the possibility of serious psychological reasons for parasomnias persisting well beyond the age at which they can usually be expected to have remitted spontaneously.

- *Nocturnal panic attacks* in children and adolescents (Garland, 1995) may not be recognized as such because of the features they share with other causes of apparently fearful behaviour at night, such as nightmares, night terrors, obstructive sleep apnoea awakenings and partial seizures.

The key features of panic attacks are a sudden awakening in a physiologically aroused state with dizziness, choking, sweating, trembling, palpitations and other distressing sensations including an intense fear of 'impending doom' (i.e. of dying). It is diagnostically helpful if panic attacks also occur during the day with other phobic symptoms, but this is not always the case. Adult studies indicate that panic attacks tend to arise from stage 2 NREM sleep. Usually, however, PSG is not necessary for differential diagnosis which essentially requires careful clinical evaluation. This is particularly important as panic attacks may coexist with other parasomnias, including arousal disorders (Garland & Smith, 1991).

There is little information about treatment. Experience with adults suggests that general anxiety-reducing methods are helpful as well as behavioural treatment and medication such as tricyclic antidepressants, selective serotonin reuptake inhibitors and benzodiazepines.

• Examples were given in the opening chapter of the many other psychiatric disorders of which sleep disturbance, including parasomnias, is a common feature. Sometimes, as in *anxiety states*, nightmares are an understandable occurrence. In *Tourette syndrome,* by contrast, the origin of the reported parasomnias is less obvious. *Sleep-related eating disorders* can be associated with daytime psychiatric disorders but, as described earlier, more usually they have been linked with a number of other sleep disorders.

In '*psychogenic dissociative states*' dramatic behaviour, sometimes bizarre or violent, is enacted at night but actually while awake (following a period of sleep) as shown by PSG. The nocturnal episodes of some patients diagnosed as having the condition began in later childhood or adolescence and are thought to have sometimes involved re-enactment of previous experiences of physical or sexual abuse (Schenck et al., 1989). Especially in young people, much care is required to distinguish between a conscious attempt to simulate a sleep disorder and a supposed limited awareness of the occurrence of such events and the reasons for them. The use of the term 'pseudoparasomnia' (Molaie & Deutsch, 1997) reflects the difficulty of making such a distinction.

Parasomnias: basic clinical approach to diagnosis

General

1 A screening question for detection of parasomnias: does the child have any unusual behaviours at night such as:

- strange sensations;
- talking, shouting, moaning or screaming;
- wandering or rushing about;
- rhythmic movements or noises;
- waking up frightened;
- wetting the bed;
- jerking of arms or legs;
- difficulty breathing;
- hurting himself.

2 Questions to be considered in describing the episodes are:
- timing;
- frequency;
- duration;
- physical and psychological features;
- level of consciousness;
- recall;
- precipitating factors.

3 Precise details are needed of sequence of subjective and objective features of episodes (including timing), ideally from the start to finish, and circumstances in which they occur. Video recordings are very helpful. Include enquiries about:
- any daytime attacks;
- neurological abnormality;
- family history.

4 Consider possible combination of different attacks, each needing separate detailed assessment.

5 Are there features to suggest the parasomnias are symptomatic of underlying psychological problem? In particular:
- frequent occurrence;
- unusually late age of onset, recurrence or persistence over many years;
- preceding trauma;
- accompanying features of psychological disorder.

6 Is there evidence of another sleep disorder of which the parasomnia is one manifestation?

Specific features

1 Occurrence in first 2 hours of overnight sleep suggests arousal disorder characterized by:
- being inaccessible during episodes;
- no recall;
- often family history.

2 Occurrence late in the night suggests REM sleep-related disorder especially:
  • true nightmares involving a frightening sequence of events (a narrative) and waking up afraid.
3 Daytime episodes when awake indicate secondary parasomnia such as:
  • epilepsy;
  • asthma;
  • panic attacks.

7

Clinical services and research

To return to the opening theme of this book, it is indefensible that sleep and its disorders feature so little in medical and other professional education and that, as a result, the standard of clinical practice is inevitably less than it ought to be. The need to correct the situation is obvious.

In fact, the need for educational improvement starts with the general public. As part of general health education it should be made clear that sleep disorders of all types are potentially harmful and that professional help for them should be sought in the expectation that effective treatment is usually possible. In order to meet raised expectations, teaching and training for those providing help will have to improve considerably. This applies to clinicians in family practice, paediatrics and child psychiatry, as well as nursing staff (especially health visitors), psychologists and also those responsible for clinical neurophysiology services. There needs to be a wider appreciation of the broad range of sleep disorders and the many treatment options rather than a preoccupation with the sleepless young child.

Provision of clinical services

Ideally, clinical services would be available at three levels.

1 Many sleep problems could be assessed and treated at the *primary care* (*general-practice*) *level*, especially the common settling and night-waking problems in toddlers (for whom help is already provided by some health visitors) and nocturnal enuresis. Some health visitors have taken the initiative and set up clinics dealing with such problems (Sykes, 1999), but such provision is geographically patchy. Also, it would be appropriate at the primary care level to more consistently include advice on a wider range of sleep disorders such as the more common parasomnias.

2 More difficult diagnostic and treatment problems would require referral to *paediatric services*, preferably working closely with *child psychiatry* for those cases where a joint approach is needed.

3 Where these measures had a limited effect, or where special diagnostic or treatment difficulties come to light, referral to a *specialized sleep disorders service* would be appropriate. Very few such centres exist. Experience in providing such a service strongly suggests that its effectiveness would be limited without wider interest and experience at the primary and secondary levels of service provision (Stores & Wiggs, 1998b). There is a basic need for a professional in the child's own locality to be responsible for co-ordinating the programme of investigation, keeping the family informed, ensuring treatment needs are met (preferably without delay) and ensuring that the child's progress is monitored in the long term.

Medical student education

Within the medical profession, promoting interest and raising standards in sleep disorders medicine should begin with undergraduates at medical school. At present, this happens only sporadically where (unusually) time has been secured in the curriculum for adequate coverage of sleep and its disorders. Recently it was shown that in the UK, out of a typical 5 year course, the median time devoted to formal medical student teaching on these topics was 5 minutes. In both the paediatric and psychiatric part of the course, the figure was 5 minutes, and, in the general practice part, zero minutes. Similar deficiencies were demonstrated for courses concerning other specialties in which patients with sleep disorders are particularly likely to be encountered (Stores & Crawford, 1998).

Comparable shortcomings have been described in North America (Rosen et al., 1993) and mainland Europe (Salzarulo, 1990). There is some recent evidence of progress in these parts of the world but, clearly, much more needs to be achieved in securing appropriate time in the undergraduate curriculum. Possible ways forward (including the exercise of political adroitness within the medical school) have been discussed by Lavie (1993).

The argument in favour of a more prominent place for sleep disorders medicine in an admittedly crowded course can easily be made on educational grounds. In 1993, the UK General Medical Council made recommendations for reorganizing medical student teaching (Education Committee of the General Medical Council, 1993). Emphasis was placed on the general themes of widespread impact of illness or disorder, integration of basic medical service and clinical issues, the inter-specialty and interdisciplinary nature of accurate diagnosis and care, and developmental aspects from infancy to old age of the nature, presentation and management of medical conditions. Sleep and its disorders lends itself particularly well to this model of teaching, not only for medical students but for other healthcare groups at various levels of training.

Specialty training

There is little reason to believe that these inadequacies in medical student teaching are corrected at postgraduate level. This is true for paediatrics and other specialities in the United States (Moline & Zendell, 1993), and there is only passing reference to sleep disorders in the UK syllabus for training in general paediatrics (Royal College of Paediatrics and Child Health, 1996). Recommended training in paediatric neurology, learning disability and clinical neurophysiology is no better in the UK regarding sleep disorders. The same is true of psychiatry, judging from recommended training at general and specialist levels and the very little mention of sleep and its disorders in examination questions. The poor representation of sleep disorders in professional teaching and training also applies to nurses (Cohen et al., 1992) and psychologists (Wiggs & Stores R., 1996; Stores R. & Wiggs, 1998), in spite of the significant part they could play in both assessment and certain forms of treatment.

Paediatric practice

In the opening chapter, examples were given of paediatric illnesses or disorders in which severe sleep disturbance of one type or another commonly occurs. Sleep can be disturbed because of the child's condition or parents' attitudes and practices, including making it especially difficult for them to impose discipline at bedtime or during the night. Alternatively, the sleep disorder may be an integral part of the illness or disorder itself. The effects of persistently disturbed sleep are likely to be serious, and the child's distress at being ill may well be made worse by the effects on mood and general well-being of not sleeping well. Parents are likely to be similarly affected.

It follows that, in a wide range of paediatric disorders, the possibility of significant sleep disturbance should be considered routinely, with a view to treating it explicitly by whatever means is appropriate, depending on the cause. This may entail advising parents about the best way to handle bedtime or waking at night; it may mean a change of treatment for the underlying physical disorder to promote more restful sleep (as in the case of asthma or epilepsy); or it may require attempts to change the child's sleep–wake cycle where the illness or disorder has led to irregular or otherwise inappropriate patterns. In these and other ways, it may be possible to improve the well-being of both child and the whole family, even where there is not much scope for fundamentally improving the underlying physical disorder. For this to be achieved, much more attention to children's sleep disorders medicine is needed in paediatrics training.

Child and adolescent psychiatry

There are many compelling reasons why psychiatrists should also be well versed in sleep disorders medicine.

As emphasized at various points earlier, *sleep disorders very commonly complicate psychiatric disorders* to an extent that is likely to exacerbate psychiatric symptoms or, at least, reduce the child's ability to cope with various difficulties.

In some instances, this *sleep disturbance may be the primary cause of the psychiatric conditions*. If this is not appreciated, treatment may be misdirected and opportunities missed to alleviate symptoms. Prominent examples of sleep disorders presenting as psychiatric disorders include the following:

- *Delayed sleep-phase syndrome* in which the physiological difficulty getting to sleep until very late, and the considerable difficulty getting up in the morning, are often misinterpreted as difficult or oppositional behaviour.
- *Upper airway obstruction* which, because of its effects on the child's quality of sleep, can produce a range of learning and behaviour problems, including ADHD symptoms.
- *Narcolepsy*, like other causes of excessive daytime sleepiness, is frequently misconstrued as laziness, other regrettable behaviour, depression or even limited intelligence. Cataplexy may be misconstrued as attention-seeking behaviour or even a conversion symptom. It has been claimed that some adults diagnosed as schizophrenic have actually been suffering from narcolepsy which only came to light when a detailed history was taken for the first time (Douglass et al., 1993). Some of these cases first showed signs of their 'psychotic' illness in adolescence. The possibility of such an error should not be overstated, but it emphasizes the importance of thorough assessment of sleep in psychiatric practice.
- *Sleep paralysis*, and other frightening sleep-related experiences, may present as anxiety or depression. The complex hallucinatory phenomena which can accompany sleep paralysis may suggest a psychotic disorder.
- The *Kleine–Levin syndrome* is commonly attributed to psychological factors because of the intermittent nature of the sleepiness, its onset following physical or psychological trauma, the often bizarre nature of the behavioural disturbance, and the hypersexuality that can accompany the periods of hypersomnia.
- *Sleepwalking and night terrors* may be thought of as psychologically determined behaviour, especially where they involve complicated behaviour (misconstrued as voluntary) or when they include acts of violence.
- *REM sleep behaviour disorder* may also be mistakenly viewed as evidence of serious psychological disturbance.
- Similarly, *parasomnias secondary to physical disorder* may well be misconstrued as psychological in origin if they take a dramatic form.

All of these conditions are likely to be further complicated psychologically by the *consequences of the sleep disorder*, such as the reactions of the child and others, limitations on school progress and social activities, and delays between the onset of symptoms and the correct diagnosis being made.

The *psychological effects of a child's sleep disorder on other members of the family* should not be overlooked. Parents may be seriously affected by worry about their child (perhaps needlessly in the absence of sound explanation or advice) or by their own persistently disrupted sleep caused by the child's sleep disturbance. Depression, impaired parent–child relationships and parenting skills, marital disharmony and underfunctioning at work are all possible consequences. Other children in the family may also suffer.

Other reasons why familiarity with sleep disorders medicine can be considered an essential part of psychiatric expertise include the possibility of sleep disturbance being an *early sign of a serious psychiatric disorder* before more definite evidence develops, and the effect of some psychotropic medications on sleep. As previously emphasized, because of the frequency with which physical illness is complicated by significant sleep disturbance, recognition and treatment of sleep disorders is a basic aspect of psychiatric liaison work with paediatrics.

Clinical research

There is a clear need for further extensive research in the field of sleep disorders medicine. Research-funding bodies share the general neglect of the field and often seem to need more than the usual amount of convincing that sleep disorders research is clinically important and relevant to large sections of the population. Where sleep disorders research is funded, there is an imbalance in favour of adult studies and, more specifically, sleep-related breathing disorders (Gillette et al., 1999). This ignores the fact that childhood sleep disorders are extremely common, very varied in nature, potentially disruptive to development in various ways, and also capable of establishing maladaptive sleep patterns persisting into adult life.

There are numerous aspects of sleep and its disorders in childhood that need to be clarified by research. The following are offered as some of the main areas where further research efforts are particularly required.

Even basic prevalence rates are not well understood. Carefully conducted *epidemiological studies* would establish the extent of sleep problems in the general population and their underlying sleep disorders. It is already clear that many children and their families affected by such disorders do not come to medical attention because the public does not consider them legitimate reasons for seeking professional help, or because they believe that no help is available. Such epidemiological research needs to be well informed about modern sleep medicine and to enquire in sufficient detail for the collected information to be meaningful. It is interesting how perfunctory enquiries about sleep have been in child health surveys which in other respects have been sophisticated. The importance of collecting information from more than one source (usually parents), as in the survey by Owens et al. (2000), was emphasized earlier. The *natural history* of children's sleep disorders is generally not well understood yet may have very practical implications. For example, is childhood OSA associated with similar problems later in life?

Similarly, well-informed surveys are needed of the *sleep disorders which commonly accompany the medical and psychiatric disorders of childhood*. It is important to clarify the extent to which sleep disturbance can add significantly to the children's difficulties and to the demands made on their parents or other carers. The point has been made already that clinical history-taking schedules, including those used in paediatrics and child psychiatry, tend to include only superficial enquiries about sleep and its disorders. Unless more appropriate enquiries are encouraged, sleep disturbance will continue often to be overlooked and its unwelcome effects ignored.

The significant *differences between sleep disorders in children and those in adults* deserves much more attention. Further clarification is needed of the many ways in which children's sleep disorders can be very different regarding their pattern of occurrence, causes, clinical manifestations, investigation and treatment needs, and natural history. Polysomnographic procedures and interpretation of the findings are often very different. Normative data for children are relatively sparse.

There would be much in favour of a *classification scheme of sleep disorders in children and adolescents* that acknowledged such differences. At present, many aspects of sleep disorders that are particularly relevant to young people have to be excavated from the essentially adult-oriented ICSD. In some instances, there is little to unearth. The section on sleep disorders associated with mental, neurological or other medical disorders in particular demonstrates the adult bias of the scheme. The restrained reference to learning disability (mental retardation) is curious in view of its strong association with sleep disturbance in people of any age affected in this way. The classification of children's sleep disorders could be acknowledged by at least an appendix to the ICSD as it stands.

The fact that *adolescence* is a time of particular risk for the development of sleep disorders, and their potentially serious complications, calls for special emphasis on this stage of development. Despite the relatively greater attention paid to sleep and its disorders at this age compared with earlier childhood, except for toddlers, many important issues remain unresolved, as emphasized by Wolfson & Carskadon (1998). These include the relative contribution to sleep changes of psychosocial and biological factors, the true extent in society of the so-called 'adolescent sleep debt' and its psychological and social consequences (including career prospects), and ways in which such complications can be avoided.

There are very obvious deficiencies in what is known about the *effects of disturbed sleep on children's cognitive function, mood and behaviour*. Experimental investigation is clearly limited by ethical constraints, but there is much scope for careful observational studies with comparisons between subjects and appropriate controls or population norms. Such psychological effects may well vary with children's age, intellectual level and also possibly sex in view of the generally greater vulnerability of boys to adverse influences on development (Kraemer, 2000).

To allow research in many of the areas to proceed, basic work is needed in the development of *further investigations suitable for use with children.*

Polysomnography services should be designed with the special needs of children and their families in mind. Preparation for recordings, the recording procedures and the overall ambience of the recording environment need to be child-friendly with technicians and other staff experienced in working with young patients. This is particularly true of laboratory PSG. Home PSG systems are generally more acceptable to children, but standardization of the procedure (including observations during the recording period) has received little attention. Normative data for home recordings (only recently available to a limited extent) have already demonstrated differences between PSG performed at home and in the laboratory setting (Stores et al., 1998a). The point has also been made earlier that diagnostic criteria based on adult studies may not apply to children in view of their physiological differences compared with older subjects.

Similarly, basic research and development is needed for *psychological measures.* Adaptation of adult scales for use with children should meet the usual psychometric requirements that they are demonstrably reliable and valid. The diversity of measures of cognitive function, mood and behaviour used in different studies of children indicates the uncertainty about appropriate and sensitive measures of the psychological effects of sleep disturbance at different ages and at different levels of ability. This is an obvious part of the sleep disorders field in which psychologists have much to contribute.

The same is true regarding the need for further studies of the various *treatments* for sleep disorders, including those of a psychological type in which psychologists should be particularly experienced. At present, there are very few results from randomized controlled or otherwise methodologically sound trials, even for settling and night-waking problems in toddlers (Mindell, 1999; Ramchandani et al., 2000). Evaluation of the range of psychological, chronobiological, pharmacological and even surgical treatments that have been described provides a rich field of opportunity for research of both clinical and theoretical appeal.

In view of the large number of children who could benefit from treatment if clinical resources were adequate, there is a need to *simplify treatment procedures* as far as possible to reduce the time and level of expertise required. A promising start has been made, for example on developing booklet forms of treatment for settling and night-waking problems in children in the general population (Scott & Richards, 1990) and also children with a learning disability (Montgomery et al.,

2000). Such methods are capable of being used to good effect by members of the primary care team, but further research is needed to identify their strengths and limitations in view of the fact that results have not always been positive, as is also the case with attempts to advise parents in groups (Owens et al., 1999a).

Needless to say, it would be highly advantageous to all concerned if sleep problems could be *prevented* in the first place. Advice (e.g. in postnatal classes) on how this might be achieved, is likely to be well received by parents (Hewitt & Galbraith, 1987). It is possible to suggest ways in which satisfactory sleep can be promoted, and the severity of certain sleep disorders lessened, by drawing on general principles such as those described earlier concerning sleep hygiene. However, there has been very little research on more specific ways in which sleep disorders might be prevented. With few exceptions (e.g. Wolfson et al., 1992; Kerr et al., 1996), this is so even for infants. Clearly, this omission needs to be corrected in view of the commonness of sleep problems at an early age, the distress they can cause within the family, and the possibility that the disturbed sleep patterns may continue in later life, with their attendant adverse psychological and social effects that were highlighted in the opening chapters.

At the outset, it was suggested that the fact that sleep disorders medicine crosses many traditional boundaries between different medical specialties and other disciplines has been a reason for its relatively slow development. It is hoped that, with advances in professional education, the essentially interdisciplinary nature of sleep disorders medicine (especially in children) will be increasingly seen as its great appeal.

Glossary

Glossary of terms used in sleep disorders medicine

This glossary is reproduced from the International Classification of Sleep Disorders – Revised (1997) with the permission of the American Academy of Sleep Medicine. The glossary in largely adult-based but, in the absence of an official version specifically concerned with children and adolescents, it is included here (in its entirety and original form) as an aid to the reader of the sleep disorders medicine literature in general, including the present book and the references cited as sources of further information.

actigraph A biomedical instrument used to measure body movement.

active sleep A term used in the phylogenetic and ontogenetic literature for the stage of sleep that is considered to be equivalent to REM (rapid eye movement) sleep. *See* REM sleep.

alpha activity An alpha electroencephalographic wave or sequence of waves with a frequency of 8 to 13 Hz.

alpha–delta sleep Sleep in which alpha activity occurs during slow wave sleep. Because alpha–delta sleep is rarely seen without alpha occurring in other sleep stages, the term alpha sleep is preferred.

alpha intrusion (-infiltration, -insertion, -interruption) A brief superimposition of electroencephalographic alpha activity on sleep activities during a stage of sleep.

alpha rhythm In human adults, an electroencephalographic rhythm with a frequency of 8 to 13 Hz, which is most prominent over the parieto-occipital cortex when the eyes are closed. The rhythm is blocked by eye opening or other arousing stimuli. It is indicative of the awake state in most normal individuals. It is most consistent and predominant during relaxed wakefulness, particularly with reduction of visual input. The amplitude is variable but typically below 50 μV in the adult. The alpha rhythm of an individual usually slows by 0.5 to 1.5 Hz and becomes more diffuse during drowsiness. The frequency range also varies with age; it is slower in children and older age groups relative to young and middle-aged adults.

alpha sleep   Sleep in which alpha activity occurs during most, if not all, sleep stages.

apnea   Cessation of airflow at the nostrils and mouth lasting at least 10 seconds. The three types of apnea are obstructive, central, and mixed. Obstructive apnea is secondary to upper-airway obstruction; central apnea is associated with a cessation of all respiratory movements; mixed apnea has both central and obstructive components.

apnea–hypopnea index   The number of apneic episodes (obstructive, central, and mixed) plus hypopneas per hour of sleep, as determined by all-night polysomnography.

apnea index   The number of apneic episodes (obstructive, central, and mixed) per hour of sleep, as determined by all-night polysomnography. A separate obstructive apnea index or central apnea index sometimes is stated.

arise time   The clock time at which an individual gets out of bed after the final awakening of the major sleep episode. This is distinguished from final wake-up.

arousal   An abrupt change from a 'deeper' stage of non-REM (NREM) sleep to a 'lighter' stage, or from REM sleep toward wakefulness, with the possibility of awakening as the final outcome. Arousal may be accompanied by increased tonic electromyographic activity and heart rate, as well as by an increased number of body movements.

arousal disorder   A parasomnia disorder presumed to be due to an abnormal arousal mechanism. Forced arousal from sleep can induce episodes. The 'classic' arousal disorders are sleepwalking, sleep terrors, and confusional arousals.

awakening   The return to the polysomnographically defined awake state from any NREM or REM sleep stages. It is characterized by alpha and beta electro-encephalographic activity, a rise in tonic electromyographic activity, voluntary rapid eye movements, and eye blinks. This definition of awakenings is valid only insofar as the polysomnogram is paralleled by a resumption of a reasonably alert state of awareness of the environment.

axial system   A means of stating different types of information in a systematic manner by listing on several 'axes', to ensure that important information is not overlooked by the statement of a single major diagnosis. *The International Classification of Sleep Disorders* uses a three-axial system: axes A, B and C.

axis A   The first level of the *International Classification of Sleep Disorders* axial system on which the sleep disorder diagnoses, modifiers, and associated code numbers are stated.

axis B   The second level of the *International Classification of Sleep Disorders* axial system on which the sleep-related procedures and procedure features, and associated code numbers, are stated.

axis C   The third level of the *International Classification of Sleep Disorders* axial system on which *ICD-9-CM* nonsleep diagnoses and associated code numbers are stated.

baseline   The typical or normal state of an individual or of an investigative variable before an experimental manipulation.

bedtime   The clock time when one attempts to fall asleep, as differentiated from the clock time when one gets into bed.

beta activity   A beta electroencephalographic wave or sequence of waves with a frequency of greater than 13 Hz.

beta rhythm   An electroencephalographic rhythm in the range of 13 to 35 Hz, when the predominant frequency, beta rhythm, is usually associated with alert wakefulness or vigilance and is accompanied by a high tonic electromyogram. The amplitude of beta rhythm is variable but usually is below 30 μV. This rhythm may be drug induced.

brain wave   Use of this term is discouraged. The suggested term is electro-encephalographic wave.

cataplexy   A sudden decrement in muscle tone and loss of deep tendon reflexes, leading to muscle weakness, paralysis or postural collapse. Cataplexy usually is precipitated by an outburst of emotional expression – notably laughter, anger or startle. One of the tetrad of symptoms of narcolepsy. During cataplexy, respiration and voluntary eye movements are not compromised.

Cheyne–Stokes respiration   A breathing pattern characterized by regular 'crescendo-decrescendo' fluctuations in respiratory rate and tidal volume.

chronobiology   The science relating to temporal, primarily rhythmic, processes in biology.

circadian rhythm   An innate daily fluctuation of physiologic or behaviour functions, including sleep–wake states, generally tied to the 24-hour daily dark–light cycle. This rhythm sometimes occurs at a measurably different periodicity (e.g. 23 or 25 hours) when light–dark and other time cues are removed.

circasemidian rhythm   A biologic rhythm that has a period length of about half a day.

conditioned insomnia   An insomnia that is produced by the development of conditioned arousal during an earlier experience of sleeplessness. Causes of the conditioned stimulus can include the customary sleep environment or thoughts of disturbed sleep. A conditioned insomnia is one component of psychophysiologic insomnia.

constant routine   A chronobiologic test of the endogenous pacemaker that involves a 36-hour baseline-monitoring period, followed by a 40-hour waking episode of monitoring with the individual on a constant routine of food intake, position, activity, and light exposure.

cycle   A characteristic of an event that exhibits rhythmic fluctuations. One cycle is defined as the activity from one maximum or minimum to the next.

deep sleep   A common term for combined NREM stage 3 and stage 4 sleep. In some sleep literature, the term deep sleep is applied to REM sleep because during REM sleep, individuals have a high awakening threshold to nonsignificant stimuli. *See* 'intermediary' sleep stage; light sleep.

delayed sleep phase   A condition that occurs when the clock hour at which sleep normally occurs is moved back in time within a given 24-hour sleep–wake cycle. This results in a temporarily displaced, that is delayed, occurrence of sleep within the 24-hour cycle. The same term denotes a circadian rhythm sleep disturbance, called the delayed sleep phase syndrome.

delta activity   Electroencephalographic activity with a frequency of less than 4 Hz (usually 0.1–3.5 Hz). In the scoring of human sleep, the minimum characteristics for scoring delta waves are conventionally 75 μV (peak-to-peak) amplitude and 0.5-second duration (2 Hz) or less.

delta sleep stage   This stage is indicative of the stage of sleep in which electroencephalographic delta waves are prevalent or predominant (sleep stages 3 and 4, respectively). *See* slow wave sleep.

diagnostic criteria   Specific criteria established in *the International Classification of Sleep Disorders* to aid in determining the unequivocal presence of a particular sleep disorder.

diurnal   Pertaining to the daytime.

drowsiness   A state of quiet wakefulness that typically occurs before sleep onset. If the eyes are closed, diffuse and slowed alpha activity usually is present, which then gives way to early features of stage 1 sleep.

duration criteria   Criteria established in the *International Classification of Sleep Disorders* for determining the duration of a particular disorder as acute, subacute, or chronic.

dyssomnia   A primary disorder of initiating and maintaining sleep or of excessive sleepiness. The dyssomnias are disorders of sleep or wakefulness *per se*; they are not a parasomnia.

early morning arousal (early a.m. arousal)   Synonymous with premature morning awakening.

electroencephalogram (EEG)   A recording of the electrical activity of the brain by means of electrodes placed on the surface of the head. With the electromyogram and electro-oculogram, the electroencephalogram is one of the three basic variables used to score sleep stages and waking. Sleep recording in humans uses surface electrodes to record potential differences between brain regions and a neutral reference point, or simply between brain regions. Either the C3 or C4 (central region) placement, according to the International 10–20 System is referentially (referred to an earlobe) recorded as the standard electrode derivation from which sleep-state scoring is performed.

electromyogram (EMG)   A recording of electrical activity from the muscular system, in sleep recording, synonymous with resting muscle activity or potential. The chin EMG, along with the electroencephalogram and electro-oculogram, is one of the three basic variables used to score sleep stages and waking. Sleep recording in humans typically uses surface electrodes to measure activity from the submental muscles. These positions reflect maximally the changes in resting activity of axial body muscles. The submental muscle EMG is tonically inhibited during REM sleep.

Electro-oculogram (EOG)   A recording of voltage changes resulting from shifts in position of the ocular globes; this is possible because each globe is a positive (anterior) and negative (posterior) dipole. Along with the electroencephalogram and the electromyogram, one of the three basic variables used to score sleep stages and waking. Sleep recording in humans uses surface electrodes placed near the eyes to record the movement (incidence, direction, and velocity) of the eye-balls. Rapid eye movements in sleep form one part of the characteristics of the REM-sleep state.

end-tidal carbon dioxide   The carbon dioxide value that is usually determined at the nares by an infra-red carbon dioxide gas analyzer. The values reflect the carbon dioxide level in alveolar or pulmonary artery blood.

entrainment   Synchronization of a biologic rhythm by a forcing stimulus such as an environmental time cue (zeitgeber). During entrainment, the frequencies of the two cycles are the same or are integral multiples of each other.

epoch   A measure of duration of the sleep recording that typically is 20 or 30 seconds in duration, depending on the paper speed of the polysomnograph, and that corresponds to one page of the polysomnogram.

excessive sleepiness (somnolence, hypersomnia, excessive daytime sleepiness)   A subjective report of difficulty in maintaining the alert awake state, usually accompanied by a rapid entrance into sleep when the person is sedentary. Excessive sleepiness may be due to an excessively deep or prolonged major sleep episode. It can be quantitatively measured by use of subjectively defined rating scales of sleepiness or physiologically measured by electrophysiologic tests such as the multiple sleep latency test (*see* MSLT). Excessive sleepiness most commonly occurs during the daytime, but it may be present at night in a person, such as a shift worker, who has the major sleep episode during the daytime.

extrinsic sleep disorders   Disorders that either originate, develop, or arise from causes outside of the body. The extrinsic sleep disorders are a subgroup of the dyssomnias.

final awakening   The amount of wakefulness that occurs after the final wake-up time until the arise time (lights on).

final wake-up   The clock time at which an individual awakens for the last time before the arise time.

first-night effect   The effect of the environment and polysomnographic-recording apparatus on the quality of the subject's sleep the first night of recording. Sleep is usually of reduced quality compared to that which would be expected in the subject's usual sleeping environment, without electrodes and other recording-procedure stimuli. The subject usually will habituate to the laboratory by the time of the second night of recording.

fragmentation (pertaining to sleep architecture)   The interruption of any stage of sleep due to the appearance of another stage or to wakefulness, leading to disrupted NREM–REM sleep cycles; this term is often used to refer to the interruption of REM sleep by movement arousals or stage 2 activity. Sleep fragmentation connotes repetitive interruptions of sleep by arousals and awakenings.

free running   A chronobiologic term that refers to the natural endogenous period of a rhythm when zeitgebers are removed. In humans, it most commonly is seen in the tendency to delay some circadian rhythms, such as the sleep–wake cycle, by approximately one hour every day; this delay occurs when a person has an impaired ability to entrain or is without time cues.

hertz (Hz)   A unit of frequency; the use of this term is preferred over the use of the synonym cycles per second (cps).

hypercapnia   Elevated carbon dioxide level in blood.

hypersomnia (excessive sleepiness)   Excessively deep or prolonged major sleep period, which may be associated with difficulty in awakening. The term is primarily used as a diagnostic term (e.g. idiopathic hypersomnia) and the term excessive sleepiness is preferred to describe the symptom.

hypnagogic   Occurrence of an event during the transition from wakefulness to sleep.

hypnagogic imagery (hallucinations)   Vivid sensory images that occur at sleep onset but are particularly vivid with sleep-onset REM periods. Hypnagogic imagery is a feature of narcolepsy, in which REM periods occur at sleep onset.

hypnagogic startle   A 'sleep start' or sudden body jerk (hypnic jerk), observed normally just at sleep onset and usually resulting, at least momentarily, in an awakening.

hypnopompic (hypnopomic)   Occurrence of an event during the transition from sleep to wakefulness at the termination of a sleep episode.

hypopnea   An episode of shallow breathing (airflow reduced by at least 50%) during sleep, lasting 10 seconds or longer, usually associated with a fall in blood oxygen saturation.

ICSD sleep code   A code number of the *International Classification of the Sleep Disorders* that refers to modifying information of a diagnosis, such as associated symptom, severity and duration of a sleep disorder.

insomnia   Difficulty in initiating or maintaining sleep. This term is employed ubiquitously to indicate any and all gradations and types of sleep loss.

'intermediary' sleep stage   A term sometimes used for NREM stage 2 sleep. *See* deep sleep; light sleep. The term is often used, especially in the French literature, for stages combining elements of stage 2 and REM sleep.

into-bed time   The clock time at which a person gets into bed. The into-bed time (IBT) will be the same as the bedtime for many people but not for those who spend time in wakeful activities in bed such as reading, before attempting to sleep.

intrinsic sleep disorders   Disorders that either originate or develop from within the body or that arise from causes within the body. The intrinsic sleep disorders are a subgroup of the dyssomnias.

K-alpha   A K-complex followed by several seconds of alpha rhythm; K-alpha is a type of microarousal.

K-complex   A sharp, biphasic electroencephalographic wave followed by a high-voltage slow wave. The complex duration is at least 0.5 seconds and may be accompanied by a sleep spindle. K complexes occur spontaneously during NREM sleep and begin and define stage 2 sleep. They are thought to be evoked responses to internal stimuli. K complexes can also be elicited during sleep by external (particularly auditory) stimuli.

light–dark cycle   The periodic pattern of light (artificial or natural) alternating with darkness.

light sleep   A common term for NREM sleep stage 1, and sometimes stage 2.

maintenance of wakefulness test (MWT)   A series of measurements of the interval from 'lights out' to sleep onset that are used in the assessment of an individual's ability to remain awake. Subjects are instructed to try to remain awake in a darkened room while in a semireclined position. Long latencies to sleep are indicative of the ability to remain awake. This test is most useful for assessing the effects of sleep disorders or of medication upon the ability to remain awake.

major sleep episode   The longest sleep episode that occurs on a daily basis. This sleep episode typically is dictated by the circadian rhythm of sleep and wakefulness; also known as the conventional or habitual time for sleeping.

microsleep   An episode lasting up to 30 seconds during which external stimuli are not perceived. The polysomnogram suddenly shifts from waking characteristics to sleep. Microsleeps are associated with excessive sleepiness and automatic behaviour.

minimal criteria   Criteria of the *International Classification of Sleep Disorders* derived from the diagnostic criteria that provide the minimum features necessary for making a particular sleep disorder diagnosis.

montage   The particular arrangement by which a number of derivations are displayed simultaneously in a polysomnogram.

movement arousal   A body movement associated with an electroencephalographic pattern of arousal or a full awakening; a sleep-scoring variable.

movement time   The term used in sleep-record scoring to denote when electroencephalographic and electro-oculographic tracings are obscured for more than half the scoring epoch because of movement. This time is only scored when the preceding and subsequent epochs are in sleep.

multiple sleep latency test (MSLT)   A series of measurements of the interval from 'lights out' to sleep onset that is used in the assessment of excessive sleepiness. Subjects are allowed a fixed number of opportunities (typically four or five) to fall asleep during their customary awake period. Excessive sleepiness is characterized by short latencies. Long latencies are helpful in distinguishing physical tiredness or fatigue from true sleepiness.

muscle tone   This term is sometimes used for resting muscle potential or resting muscle activity. *See* electromyograph (EMG).

myoclonus   Muscle contractions in the form of abrupt 'jerks' or twitches that generally last less than 100 milliseconds. The term should not be applied to the periodic leg movements of sleep that characteristically have a duration of 0.5 to 5 seconds.

nap   A short sleep episode that may be intentionally or unintentionally taken during the major episode of habitual wakefulness.

nightmare   This term is used to denote an unpleasant and frightening dream that usually occurs in REM sleep. Nightmares are occasionally called dream anxiety attacks and are distinguished from sleep (night) terrors. In the past, the term nightmare has been used to indicate both sleep terrors and dream anxiety attacks.

nocturnal confusion   Episodes of delirium and disorientation that occur close to or during night-time sleep; nocturnal confusion is often seen in the elderly and is indicative of organic central nervous system deterioration.

nocturnal dyspnea   Respiratory distress that may be minimal during the day but becomes quite pronounced during sleep.

nocturnal penile tumescence (NPT)   The natural periodic cycle of penile erections that occur during sleep, typically associated with REM sleep. The preferred term is sleep-related erections.

nocturnal sleep   This term is synonymous with the typical 'night-time' or major sleep episode related to the circadian rhythm of sleep and wakefulness; it is also known as the conventional or habitual time for sleeping.

non-rapid eye movement (NREM, nonREM) sleep   *See* sleep stages.

NREM–REM sleep cycle (synonymous with sleep cycle)   A period during sleep composed of a NREM sleep episode and the subsequent REM sleep episode; each NREM–REM sleep couplet is equal to one cycle. Any NREM sleep stage suffices as the NREM sleep portion of a cycle. An adult sleep period of 6.5 to 8.5 hours generally consists of four to six cycles. The cycle duration increases from infancy to young adulthood.

NREM sleep intrusion   An interposition of NREM sleep, or a component of NREM sleep physiology (e.g. elevated electromyographic activity, K complex, sleep spindle, delta waves), in REM sleep; a portion of NREM sleep not appearing in its usual sleep-cycle position.

NREM sleep period   The NREM sleep portion of NREM–REM sleep cycle; such an episode consists primarily of sleep stages 3 and 4 early in the night and of sleep stage 2 later in the night. *See* sleep cycle; sleep stages.

obesity–hypoventilation syndrome   A term applied to obese individuals who hypoventilate during wakefulness. Because the term can apply to several different disorders, its use is discouraged.

paradoxical sleep   This term is synonymous with REM sleep, which is the preferred term.

parasomnia   A disorder of arousal, partial arousal or sleep-stage transition. It represents an episodic disorder in sleep (such as sleepwalking) rather than a disorder in the quantity or timing of sleep or wakefulness *per se*. A parasomnia may be induced or exacerbated by sleep; a parasomnia is not a dyssomnia.

paroxysm   Phenomenon of abrupt onset that rapidly attains a maximum level and terminates suddenly; paroxysm is distinguished from background activity. This term commonly refers to an epileptiform discharge on the electro-encephalogram.

paroxysmal nocturnal dyspnea (PND)   Respiratory distress and shortness of breath that are due to pulmonary edema; the dyspnea appears suddenly and often awakens the sleeping individual.

penile buckling pressure   The amount of force applied to the glans of the penis that is sufficient to produce at least a 30° bend in the shaft.

penile rigidity   The firmness of the penis as measured by the penile-buckling pressure. Normally, the fully erect penis has maximum rigidity.

period   The interval in time between the recurrence of a defined phase or moment of a rhythmic or periodic event. The time that occurs between one peak or trough and the next.

periodic leg movement (PLM)   A rapid partial flexion of the foot at the ankle, extension of the big toe, and partial flexion of the knee and hip that occurs during sleep. The movements occur with a periodicity of 20 to 60 seconds in a stereotyped pattern, lasting 0.5 to 5 seconds. PLMs are a characteristic feature of the periodic limb movement disorder.

periodic movements of sleep (PMS)   *See* periodic leg movement.

phase advance   The shift of an episode of sleep or wake to an earlier position in the 24-hour sleep–wake cycle. A shift of sleep from 11 p.m.–7 a.m. to 8 p.m.–4 a.m. represents a three-hour phase advance. *See* phase delay.

phase delay   A shift of an episode of sleep or wake to a later position of the 24-hour sleep–wake cycle. A shift of sleep from 11 p.m.–7 a.m. to 2 a.m.–10 a.m. represents a three-hour phase delay. *See* phase advance.

phase transition   One of the two junctures of the major sleep and wake phases in the 24-hour sleep–wake cycle.

phasic event (activity)   Brain, muscle, or autonomic events of a brief and episodic nature that occur in sleep; a phasic event (such as eye movements or muscle twitches) is a characteristic of REM sleep; the usual duration is milliseconds to one to two seconds.

photoperiod   The duration of light in a light–dark cycle.

Pickwickian   A term applied to an individual who snores, is obese and sleepy, and has alveolar hypoventilation. The term has been applied to many different disorders and, therefore, its use is discouraged.

PLM-arousal index   The number of sleep-related periodic leg movements per hour of sleep that are associated with an electroencephalographic arousal. *See* periodic leg movement.

PLM index   The number of periodic leg movements per hour of total sleep time as determined by all-night polysomnography; the index is sometimes expressed as the number of movements per hour of NREM sleep because the movements are usually inhibited during REM sleep. *See* periodic leg movement.

PLM percentage   The percentage of total sleep time occupied with recurrent episodes of periodic leg movements.

polysomnogram   The continuous and simultaneous recording of multiple physiologic variables during sleep, i.e. electroencephalogram, electro-oculo-gram, electromyogram (these are the three basic stage-scoring parameters), electrocardiogram, respiratory air flow, respiratory movements, leg movements and other electrophysiologic variables.

polysomnograph   A biomedical instrument used to measure physiologic variables of sleep.

polysomnographic (as in recording, monitoring, registration or tracings)   Describes a recording on paper, computer disc, or tape of a polysomnogram.

premature morning awakening (early morning awakening)   Early termination of the sleep episode, accompanied by an inability to return to sleep, sometimes after the last of several awakenings. It reflects interference at the end rather than at the commencement of the sleep episode. This awakening is a characteristic sleep disturbance of some people with depression.

proposed sleep disorder   A disorder in which insufficient information is available in the medical literature to confirm the unequivocal existence of the disorder. This is a category of the International Classification of Sleep Disorders.

quiet sleep   A term used for describing NREM sleep in infants and animals when specific NREM sleep stages 1 to 4 cannot be determined.

rapid eye movement sleep (REM sleep)   *See* sleep stages.

record   The end product of the polysomnograph recording process.

recording   The process of obtaining a polysomnographic record. The term is also applied to the end product of the polysomnograph recording process.

REM density (-intensity)   A function that expresses the frequency of eye movements per unit of time during sleep stage REM.

REM sleep episode   The REM sleep portion of a NREM–REM sleep cycle; early in the night it may be as short as 30 seconds, whereas, in later cycles, it may be longer than an hour. *See* sleep stage REM.

REM sleep intrusion   A brief interval of REM sleep appearing out of its usual position in the NREM–REM sleep cycle; an interposition of REM sleep in NREM sleep; the intrusion can sometimes be the appearance of a single, dissociated component of REM sleep (e.g. eye movements, 'drop out' of muscle tone) rather than all REM sleep parameters.

REM sleep latency   The interval from sleep onset to the first appearance of stage REM sleep in the sleep episode.

REM sleep onset   The designation for commencement of a REM sleep episode. This term can sometimes be used as a shorthand term for a sleep-onset REM-sleep episode. *See* sleep onset; sleep-onset REM period (SOREMP).

REM sleep percent   The proportion of total sleep time constituted by the REM stage of sleep.

REM sleep rebound (recovery)   The lengthening and increase in frequency and density of REM sleep episodes, which result in an increase in REM sleep percent above baseline. REM sleep rebound follows REM sleep deprivation once the depriving influence is removed.

respiratory-disturbance index (RDI) (apnea–hypopnea index)   The number of apneas (obstructive, central, or mixed) plus hypopneas per hour of total sleep time, as determined by all-night polysomnography.

restlessness (referring to a quality of sleep)   Persistent or recurrent body movements, arousals, and brief awakenings that occur in the course of sleep.

rhythm   An event that occurs at an approximately constant period length.

saw-tooth waves   A form of theta rhythm that occurs during REM sleep and is characterized by a notched appearance in the waveform. The waves occur in bursts that last up to 10 seconds.

severity criteria   Criteria for establishing the severity of a particular sleep disorder, according to the following categories: mild, moderate, or severe.

sleep architecture   The NREM–REM sleep-stage and cycle infrastructure of sleep understood from the vantage point of the quantitative relationship of these components to each other. Often plotted in the form of a histogram.

sleep cycle   Synonymous with the NREM–REM sleep cycle.

sleep efficiency (or sleep-efficiency index)   The proportion of sleep in the episode potentially filled by sleep (i.e. the ratio of total sleep time to time in bed).

sleep episode   An interval of sleep that may be voluntary or involuntary. In the sleep laboratory, the sleep episode occurs from the time of 'lights out' to the time of 'lights on'. The major sleep episode is usually the longest daily sleep episode.

sleep hygiene   The conditions and practices that promote continuous and effective sleep. These include regularity of bedtime and arise time; conformity of time spent in bed to the time necessary for sustained and individually adequate sleep (i.e. the total sleep time sufficient to avoid sleepiness when awake); restriction of alcohol and caffeine beverages before bedtime; and employment of exercise, nutrition and environment factors so that they enhance, not disturb, restful sleep.

sleepiness (somnolence, drowsiness)   Difficulty in maintaining alert wakefulness so that the person falls asleep if not actively kept aroused. The sleepiness is not simply a feeling of physical tiredness or listlessness. When sleepiness occurs in inappropriate circumstances, it is considered to be excessive sleepiness.

sleep interruption   Breaks in sleep that result in arousal and wakefulness. *See* fragmentation; restlessness.

sleep latency   The duration of time from 'lights out', or bedtime, to the onset of sleep.

sleep log (diary)   A daily, written record of a person's sleep–wake pattern that contains such information as time of retiring and arising, time in bed, estimated total sleep time, number and duration of sleep interruptions, quality of sleep, daytime naps, use of medications or caffeine-containing beverages, and the nature of waking activities.

sleep maintenance DIMS (insomnia)   A disturbance in maintaining sleep after sleep onset is achieved; persistently interrupted sleep without difficulty falling asleep; a disorder characterized by sleep-continuity disturbance.

sleep mentation   The imagery and thinking experienced during sleep. Sleep mentation usually consists of combinations of images and thoughts during REM sleep. Imagery is vividly expressed in dreams involving all the senses in approximate proportion to their waking representations. Mentation is experienced generally less distinctly in NREM sleep, but it may be quite vivid in stage 2 sleep, especially towards the end of the sleep episode. Mentation at sleep onset (hypnagogic reverie) can be as vivid as that which occurs during REM sleep.

sleep onset   The transition from awake to sleep, normally to NREM stage 1 sleep but in certain conditions, such as infancy and narcolepsy, into stage REM sleep. To establish sleep onset, most polysomnographers accept electro-encephalographic slowing, reduction and eventual disappearance of alpha activity, presence of electroencephalographic vertex sharp transients, and slow rolling eye movements (the components of NREM stage 1) as sufficient for sleep onset; others require appearance of stage 2 patterns. *See* latency; sleep stages.

sleep-onset REM period (SOREMP)   The beginning of sleep by entrance directly into stage REM sleep. The onset of REM sleep occurs within 10 minutes of sleep onset.

sleep paralysis   Immobility of the body that occurs in the transition from sleep to wakefulness (i.e. atonia); this is a partial manifestation of REM sleep.

sleep pattern (24-hour sleep–wake pattern)   A person's clock-hour schedule of bedtime and arise time as well as nap behaviour; the sleep pattern may also include time and duration of sleep interruptions. *See* sleep–wake cycle; circadian rhythm; sleep log.

sleep-related erections   The natural periodic cycle of penile erections that occur during sleep, typically associated with REM sleep. Sleep-related erectile activity can be characterized by four phases: T-up (ascending tumescence), T-max (plateau maximal tumescence), T-down (detumescence), and T-zero (no tumescence). Polysomnographic assessment of sleep-related erections is useful for differentiating organic from nonorganic erectile dysfunction.

sleep spindle   Spindle-shaped bursts of 11.5- to 15-HZ electroencephalographic waveforms that last 0.5 to 1.5 seconds. The spindle bursts are generally diffuse, but they are of highest voltage over the central regions of the head. The amplitude is generally less than 50 μV in the adult. These waveforms are one of the identifying electroencephalographic features of NREM stage 2 sleep; they may persist into NREM stages 3 and 4 but generally are not seen in REM sleep.

sleep stage demarcation   The significant polysomnographic characteristics that distinguish the boundaries of the sleep stages. In certain conditions and with the use of certain drugs, sleep stage demarcations may be blurred or lost, making it difficult to identify certain stages with certainty or to distinguish the temporal limits of sleep stage lengths.

sleep stage episode   A sleep stage interval that represents the stage in a NREM–REM sleep cycle; this concept is easiest to comprehend in relation to REM sleep, which is a homogeneous stage, i.e. the fourth REM sleep episode is in the fourth sleep cycle (unless a prior REM episode was skipped). If one interval of REM sleep is separated from another by more than 20 minutes, they constitute separate REM sleep episodes (and are in separate sleep cycles); a sleep stage episode may be of any duration.

sleep stage NREM   One of the two major sleep states, distinguished from REM sleep; this stage comprises sleep stages 1 to 4, which constitute levels in the spectrum of NREM sleep 'depth' or physiologic intensity.

sleep stage REM   The stage of sleep with the highest brain activity, characterized by enhanced brain metabolism and vivid hallucinatory imagery or dreaming. There are spontaneous rapid eye movements, resting muscle activity is suppressed, and awakening threshold to nonsignificant stimuli is high. The electroencephalogram is a low-voltage, mixed-frequency, nonalpha record. REM sleep is usually 20% to 25% of total sleep time. It is also called 'paradoxical sleep'.

sleep stages   Distinctive stages of sleep, best demonstrated by polysomnographic recordings of the electroencephalogram, electro-oculogram, and electromyogram.

sleep stage 1 (NREM stage 1)   A stage of NREM sleep that occurs at sleep onset or that follows arousal from sleep stages 2, 3, 4 or REM. It consists of a relatively low-voltage electroencephalographic recording with mixed frequency, mainly theta activity, and alpha activity of less than 50% of the scoring epoch. It contains electroencephalographic vertex waves and slow rolling eye movements and no sleep spindles, K complexes or REMs. Stage 1 sleep normally represents 4% to 5% of the major sleep episode.

sleep stage 2 (NREM stage 2)   A stage of NREM sleep characterized by the presence of sleep spindles and K complexes present in a relatively low-voltage, mixed-frequency electroencephalographic background; high-voltage delta waves may comprise up to 20% of stage 2 epochs. Stage 2 sleep usually accounts for 45% to 55% of the major sleep episode.

sleep stage 3 (NREM stage 3)   A stage of NREM sleep defined by at least 20% and not more than 50% of the episode consisting of electroencephalographic waves less than 2 Hz and more than 75 µV (high-amplitude delta waves). This is also known as a 'delta' sleep stage. In combination with stage 4, it constitutes 'deep' NREM sleep or slow wave sleep; this stage is often combined with stage 4 into NREM sleep stage 3/4 because of the lack of documented physiologic differences between the two stages. Stage 3 sleep usually appears only in the first third of the sleep episode and usually comprises 4% to 6% of total sleep time.

sleep stage 4 (NREM stage 4)   All statements concerning NREM sleep stage 3 apply to sleep stage 4 except that high-voltage, electroencephalographic slow waves persist during 50% or more of the epoch in stage 4 sleep. NREM sleep stage 4 usually represents 12% to 15% of the total sleep time. Sleepwalking, sleep terrors, and confusional–arousal episodes generally begin in stage 4 or during arousals from this stage. *See* sleep stage 3.

sleep structure   This term refers to sleep architecture. In addition to encompassing sleep stages and sleep cycle relationships, however, sleep structure assesses the within-stage qualities of the electroencephalogram and other physiologic attributes.

sleep talking   Talking in sleep that usually occurs in the course of transitory arousals from NREM sleep. The talking can occur during stage REM sleep, at which time it represents a motor breakthrough of dream speech. Full consciousness is not achieved, and no memory of the event remains.

sleep–wake cycle   Basically, the clock-hour relationships of the major sleep and wake episodes in the 24-hour cycle. *See* phase transition; circadian rhythm.

sleep–wake shift (change, reversal)   A shift that occurs when sleep as a whole, or in part, is moved to a time of customary waking activity, and the latter is moved to the time of the major sleep episode. This shift is common during periods of jet lag and shift work.

sleep–wake transition disorder   A disorder that occurs during the transition from wakefulness to sleep or from one sleep stage to another. This disorder is a form of the parasomnias and is not a dyssomnia.

slow wave sleep (SWS)   Sleep characterized by electroencephalographic waves of duration slower than 8 Hz. This term is synonymous with sleep stages 3 plus 4 combined. *See* delta sleep stage.

snoring   A noise produced primarily with inspiratory respiration during sleep that is due to vibration of the soft palate and the pillars of the oropharyngeal inlet. All snorers have incomplete obstruction of the upper-airway, and many habitual snorers have complete episodes of upper-airway obstruction.

spindle REM sleep   A condition in which sleep spindles persist atypically in REM sleep; this finding is seen in patients with chronic insomnia conditions and occasionally in the first REM period.

synchronized   A chronobiologic term used to indicate that two or more rhythms recur with the same phase relationship. In electroencephalography it is used to indicate an increased amplitude and usually a decreased frequency of the dominant activities.

theta activity   Electroencephalographic activity with a frequency of 4 to 8 Hz, generally maximal over the central and temporal cortex.

total recording time (TRT)   The duration of time from sleep onset to final awakening. In addition to total sleep time, it comprises the time taken up by wake periods and movement time until final awakening. *See* sleep efficiency.

total sleep episode   This is the total time available for sleep during an attempt to sleep. It comprises NREM and REM sleep, as well as wakefulness. This term is synonymous with and preferred to the term total sleep period.

total sleep time (TST)   The amount of actual sleep time in a sleep episode; this time is equal to the total sleep episode less the awake time. Total sleep time is the total of all REM and NREM sleep in a sleep episode.

trace alternant   An electroencephalographic pattern of sleeping newborns, characterized by bursts of slow waves, at times intermixed with sharp waves, and intervening periods of relative quiescence with extreme low-amplitude activity.

tumescence (penile)   Hardening and expansion of the penis (penile erection). When associated with REM sleep, it is referred to as a sleep-related erection.

twitch (body twitch)   A very small body movement such as a local foot or finger jerk; this movement usually is not associated with arousal.

vertex sharp transient   Sharp negative potential, maximal at the vertex, occurring spontaneously during sleep or in response to a sensory stimulus during sleep or wakefulness. The amplitude varies but rarely exceeds 250 μV. Use of the term vertex sharp wave is discouraged.

wake time   The total time occurring between sleep onset and final wake-up time that is scored as wakefulness in a polysomnogram.

waxing and waning   A crescendo–decrescendo pattern of activity, usually electroencephalographic activity.

zeitgeber   An environmental time cue, such as sunlight, noise, social interaction, alarm clocks, that usually helps an individual entrain to the 24-hour day.

List of abbreviations

AHI	Apnea–Hypopnea Index
AI	Aapnea Index
ASDA	American Sleep Disorders Association
CNS	Central Nervous System
DIMS	Disorder of Initiating and Maintaining Sleep
DOES	Disorders of Excessive Somnolence
DSM	Diagnostic and Statistical Manual
EEG	Electroencephalogram
EMG	Electromyogram

EOG	Electrooculogram
Hz	Hertz (cycles per second)
ICD	International Classification of Diseases
ICSD	International Classification of Sleep Disorders
MSLT	Multiple Sleep Latency Test
MWT	Maintenance of Wakefulness Test
NPT	Nocturnal Penile Tumescence
NOS	Not Otherwise Specified
NREM	Nonrapid Eye Movement (sleep)
PLM	Periodic Leg Movement
PND	Paroxysmal Nocturnal Dystonia
PSG	Polysomnogram
RDI	Pespiratory-Disturbance Index
REM	Rapid Eye Movement (sleep)
REMs	Rapid Eye Movements
RLS	Restless Legs Syndrome
SDB	Sleep-Disordered Breathing
SOREMP	Sleep-Onset REM Period
SWS	Slow Wave Sleep
TST	Total Sleep Time

References

Acebo, C., Sadeh, A., Seifer, R., Tzischinsky, O., Wolfson, A. R., Hafer, A. & Carskadon, M. A. (1999). Estimating sleep patterns with activity monitoring in children and adolescents: How many nights are necessary for reliable measures? *Sleep*, **22**, 95–103.

Adair, R., Bauchner, H., Philipp, B., Levenson, S. & Zuckerman, B. (1991). Night waking during infancy: role of parental presence at bedtime. *Pediatrics*, **84**, 500–4.

Adam, K. & Oswald, I. (1984). Sleep helps healing. *British Medical Journal*, **289**, 1400–1.

Akerstedt, T. (1998). Shift work and disturbed sleep/wakefulness. *Sleep Medicine Reviews*, **2**, 117–28.

American Sleep Disorders Association (1992). The clinical use of the Multiple Sleep Latency Test. *Sleep*, **15**, 268–76.

American Sleep Disorders Association (1995). The role of actigraphy in the evaluation of sleep disorders. *Sleep*, **18**, 288–302.

American Sleep Disorders Association (1997). *ICSD – International Classification of Sleep Disorders, Revised: Diagnostic and Coding Manual*. American Sleep Disorders Association.

American Thoracic Society (1996). Standards and indicators for cardiopulmonary sleep studies in children. *American Journal of Respiratory and Critical Care Medicine*, **153**, 866–78.

Anders, T., Emde, R. & Parmelee, A. (eds.) (1971). *A Manual of Standardised Terminology, Techniques and Criteria for the Scoring of States of Sleep and Wakefulness in Newborn Infants*. Los Angeles: UCLA Brain Information Services.

Anders, T. F., Carskadon, M. A., Dement, W. C. & Harvey, K. (1978). Sleep habits of children and the identification of pathologically sleepy children. *Child Psychiatry and Human Development*, **9**, 56–63.

Arens, R., Wright, B., Elliot, J., Zhao, H., Wang, P. P., Brown, L. W., Namey, T. & Kaplan, P. (1998). Periodic limb movement in sleep in children with Williams syndrome. *Journal of Pediatrics*, **133**, 670–4.

Armstrong, K. L., O'Donnell, H., McCallum, R. & Dadds, M. (1998). Childhood sleep problems: association with prenatal factors and maternal distress/depression. *Journal of Pediatrics and Child Health*, **34**, 263–6.

Aserinsky, E. & Kleitman, N. (1953). Regularly occurring periods of eye motility, and concomitant phenomena, during sleep. *Science*, **118**, 273–4.

Atar, D., Lehman, W. B. & Grant, A. D. (1991). Growing pains. *Orthopaedic Review*, **20**, 133–6.

Attarian, H. (2000). Sleep and neuromuscular disorders. *Sleep Medicine*, **1**, 3–9.

Autret, A., de Toffo, I. B., Corcia, Ph., Uommet, C., Prunier-Levilion, C. & Lucas, B. (1999). Sleep and epilepsy. *Sleep Medicine Reviews*, **3**, 201–17.

Avital, A., Steljes, D. G., Pasterkamp, H., Kryger, M., Sanchez, I. & Chernick, V. (1991). Sleep quality in children with asthma treated with theophylline or cromolyn sodium. *Journal of Pediatrics*, **119**, 979–84.

Bader, G. & Lavigne, G. (2000). Sleep bruxism; an overview of an oromandibular sleep movement disorder. *Sleep Medicine Reviews*, **4**, 27–43.

Ball, J. & Koloian, B. (1995). Sleep patterns among ADHD children. *Clinical Psychology Review*, **15**, 681–91.

Barabas, G., Ferrari, M., Schemp, P. & Matthews, W. S. (1983). Childhood migraine and somnambulism. *Neurology*, **33**, 945–9.

Bassetti, C. & Aldrich, M. S. (2000). Narcolepsy, idiopathic hypersomnia and periodic hypersomnias. In *Sleep Disorders in Neurological Disease*, ed. A. Culebras, pp. 323–54, New York: Marcel Dekker.

Bax, M. & Colville, G. A. (1995). Behaviour in mucopolysaccharide disorders. *Archives of Disease in Childhood*, **73**, 77–81.

Benca, R. M. & Casper, R. C. (2000). Eating disorders. In *Principles and Practice of Sleep Medicine*, 3rd edn, ed. M. H. Kryger, T. Roth & W. C. Dement, pp. 1169–75, Philadelphia: Saunders.

Billiard, M. (1996). Idiopathic hypersomnia. *Neurologic Clinics*, **14**, 573–82.

Billiard, M., Guilleminault, C. & Dement, W. (1975). A menstrual linked periodic hypersomnia. *Neurology*, **25**, 436–43.

Billiard, M., Alperovitch, A., Perot, C. & Jammes, A. (1987). Excessive daytime somnolence in young men: prevalence and contributing factors. *Sleep*, **10**, 297–305.

Blatt, I., Peled, R., Gadoth, N. & Lavie, P. (1991). The value of sleep recording in evaluating somnambulism in young adults. *Electroencephalography and Clinical Neurophysiology*, **78**, 407–13.

Blum, N. J. (1999). Severe sleep problems among infants. *Acta Paediatrica*, **88**, 1318–19.

Bonnet, M. H. (2000). Sleep deprivation. In *Principles and Practice of Sleep Medicine*, 3rd edn, ed. M. H. Kryger, T. Roth & W. C. Dement, pp. 53–71, Philadelphia: Saunders.

Bonnet, M. H. & Arand, D. L. (1995). We are chronically sleep deprived. *Sleep*, **18**, 908–11.

Boselli, M., Parrino, L., Smerieri, A. & Terzano, M. G. (1998). Effect of age on EEG arousals in normal sleep. *Sleep*, **21**, 351–7.

Breslau, N., Roth, T., Rosenthal, L. & Andreski, P. (1996). Sleep disturbance and psychiatric disorders: a longitudinal epidemiological study of young adults. *Biological Psychiatry*, **39**, 411–18.

Brockhaus, A. & Elger, C. E. (1995). Complex partial seizures of temporal lobe origin in children of different age groups. *Epilepsia*, **36**, 1173–81.

Broughton, R. J. (1999). Polysomnography: Principles and applications in sleep and arousal disorders. In *Electroencephalography: Basic Principles, Clinical Applications and Related Fields*, 4th edn, ed. E. Niedermeyer & F. Lopes da Silva, pp. 858–95. Baltimore: Williams & Wilkins.

Broughton, R., Billings, R., Cartwright, R. et al. (1994). Homicidal somnambulism: A case report. *Sleep*, **1**, 253–64.

Broughton, R. J. & Shimizu, T. (1997). Dangerous behaviours by night. In *Forensic Aspects of Sleep*, ed. C. Shapiro & A. McCall Smith, pp. 65–83, Chichester: Wiley.

Brouillette, R. T., Morielli, A., Leimanis, A. et al. (2000). Nocturnal pulse oximetry as an abbreviated test modality for pediatric obstructive sleep apnea. *Pediatrics*, **105**, 405–12.

Bruni, O., Ottaviano, S., Guidetti, V. et al. (1996). The Sleep Disturbance Scale for Children (SDSC). Construction and validation of an instrument to evaluate sleep disturbances in childhood and adolescence. *Journal of Sleep Research*, **5**, 251–61.

Burton, A. (1990). The management of sleep problems. In *Profound Retardation and Multiple Impairment*. Vol. 3, *Medical and Physical Care and Management*, ed. J. Hogg, J. Sebba & I. Lambe, pp. 274–84. London: Chapman and Hall.

Canivet, C., Jakobsson, I. & Hagander, B. (2000). Infantile colic. Follow up at four years of age: still more 'emotional'. *Acta Paediatrica*, **89**, 13–17.

Carroll, J. L. (1996). Sleep-related upper airway obstruction in children and adolescents. *Child and Adolescent Psychiatric Clinics of North America*, **5**, 617–47.

Carroll, J. L. & Loughlin, G. M. (1995a). Primary snoring in children. In *Principles and Practice of Sleep Medicine in the Child*, ed. R. Ferber & M. Kryger, pp. 155–11. Philadelphia: Saunders.

Carroll, J. L. & Loughlin, G. M. (1995b). Obstructive sleep apnea syndrome in infants and children: diagnosis and management. In *Principles and Practice of Sleep Medicine in the Child*, ed. R. Ferber & M. Kryger, pp. 193–216. Philadelphia: Saunders.

Carroll, J. L. & Loughlin, G. M. (1995c). Obstructive sleep apnoea syndrome in infants and children: clinical features and pathophysiology. In *Principles and Practice of Sleep Medicine in the Child*, ed. R. Ferber & M. Kryger, pp. 163–91. Philadelphia: Saunders.

Carroll, J. L., McColley, S. A., Marcus, C. L., Curtis, S. & Loughlin, G. M. (1995). Inability of clinical history to distinguish primary snoring from obstructive sleep apnea in children. *Chest*, **108**, 610–18.

Carskadon, M. A. (1990). Adolescent sleepiness: increased risk in a high risk population. *Alcohol, Drugs and Driving*, **5/6**, 317–27.

Carskadon, M. & Dement, W. C. (1981). Cumulative effects of sleep restriction on daytime sleepiness. *Psychophysiology*, **18**, 107–18.

Carskadon, M. A. & Dement, W. C. (1987). Sleepiness in the normal adolescent. In *Sleep and its Disorders in Children*, ed. C. Guilleminault, pp. 53–66. New York: Raven Press.

Carskadon, M. A., Acebo, C., Richardson, G. S., Tate, B. A. & Seifer, R. (1997). Long nights protocol: access to circadian parameters in adolescents. *Journal of Biological Rhythms*, **12**, 278–89.

Cavallo, A. (1992). Plasma melatonin rhythm in normal puberty: interactions of age and pubertal states. *Neuroendocrinology*, **55**, 372–9.

Challamel, M.-J. & Cochat, P. (1999). Enuresis: pathophysiology and treatment. *Sleep Medicine Reviews*, **3**, 313–24.

Challamel, M.-J., Mazzola, M.-E., Nevsimalova, S., Cannard, C., Louis, J. & Revol, M. (1994). Narcolepsy in children. *Sleep*, **17**, supplement S17–S20.

Chatoor, I., Wells, K. C., Connors, C. K., Seidel, W. T. & Shaw, D. (1983). The effects of nocturnally administered stimulant medication on EEG, sleep and behavior in hyperactive children. *Journal of the American Academy of Child Psychiatry*, **22**, 337–42.

Chavin, W. & Tinson, S. (1980). Children with sleep difficulties. *Health Visitor*, **53**, 477–80.

Chervin, R. D., Dillon, J. E., Bassetti, C., Ganoczy, D. A. & Pituch, K. J. (1997). Symptoms of sleep disorders, inattention and hyperactivity in children. *Sleep*, **20**, 1185–92.

Chervin, R. D., Hedger, K., Dillon, J. E. & Pituch, K. J. (2000). Pediatric Sleep Questionnaire (PSQ): Validity and reliability of scales for sleep-disordered breathing, snoring, sleepiness, and behavioral problems. *Sleep Medicine*, **1**, 21–32.

Chesson, A. L., Littner, M., Davila, D. et al. (1999a). Practice parameters for the use of light therapy in the treatment of sleep disorders. *Sleep*, **22**, 641–8.

Chesson, A. L., Wise, M., Davila, D. et al. (1999b). Practice parameters for the treatment of restless legs syndrome and periodic limb movement disorder. *Sleep*, **22**, 961–8.

Cirignotta, F., Zucconi, M., Mondini, S., Gerardi, R. & Lugaresi, E. (1989). Cerebral anoxic attacks in sleep apnea syndrome. *Sleep*, **12**, 400–4.

Clayton-Smith, J. (1993). Clinical research on Angelman syndrome in the United Kingdom: observations on 82 affected individuals. *American Journal of Medical Genetics*, **46**, 12–15.

Clift, S., Dahlitz, M. & Parkes, J. D. (1994). Sleep apnoea in the Prader–Willi syndrome. *Journal of Sleep Research*, **3**, 121–6.

Cohen, F. L., Merritt, S. L., Nehring, W. M., Mercer, P. W. & Eshler, B. C. (1992). Curricular sleep content in graduate and undergraduate nursing programs. *Sleep Research*, **21**, 187.

Colley, A. F., Leversha, M. A., Voullaire, L. E. & Rogers, J. G. (1990). Five cases demonstrating the distinctive behavioural features of chromosome deletion 17 (p 11.2 p 11.2) (Smith–Magenis syndrome). *Journal of Paediatrics and Child Health*, **26**, 17–21.

Commission on Classification and Terminology of the International League Against Epilepsy (1989). Proposal for revised classification of epilepsies and epileptic syndromes. *Epilepsia*, **30**, 389–99.

Corbo, G. M., Fuciarelli, F., Foresi, A. & De-Benedetto, F. (1989). Snoring in children: association with respiratory symptoms and passive smoking. *British Medical Journal*, **299**, 1491–4 (published erratum British Medical Journal, 1990, **300**, 226).

Corkum, P., Tannock, R. & Moldofsky, H. (1998). Sleep disturbances in children with attention-deficit/hyperactivity disorder. *Journal of the American Academy of Child and Adolescent Psychiatry*, **37**, 637–46.

Cornwell, A. C. (1995). Sleep and sudden infant death syndrome. In *Clinical Handbook of Sleep Disorders in Children*, ed. C. E. Schaefer, pp. 15–47. Northvale NJ: Jason Aronson.

Cortesi, G., Giannotti, F. & Ottaviano, S. (1999). Sleep problems and daytime behaviour in childhood idiopathic epilepsy. *Epilepsia*, **40**, 1557–65.

Cosnett, J. E. (1992). Charles Dickens: observer of sleep and its disorders. *Sleep*, **15**, 264–7.

Cureton-Lane, R. A. & Fontaine, D. K. (1997). Sleep in the pediatric ICU: an empirical investigation. *American Journal of Critical Care*, **6**, 56–63.

Czeisler, C. A., Richardson, G. S., Coleman, R. M. et al. (1981). Chronotherapy: resetting the circadian clock of patients with delayed sleep insomnia. *Sleep*, **4**, 1–21.

Czeisler, C. A., Shanahan, T. L., Klerman, E. B. et al. (1995). Suppression of melatonin secretion in some blind patients by exposure to bright light. *New Zealand Journal of Medicine*, **332**, 6–11.

Czeisler, C. A., Duffy, J. F., Shanahan, T. L. et al. (1999). Stability, precision and near 24 hour period of the human circadian pacemaker. *Science*, **284**, 2177–81.

Dahl, R. E. (1996a). The impact of inadequate sleep on children's daytime cognitive function. *Seminars in Pediatric Neurology*, **3**, 44–50.

Dahl, R. E. (1996b). Narcolepsy in children and adolescents. *Child and Adolescent Psychiatric Clinics of North America*, **5**, 649–59.

Dahl, R. E. & Puig-Antich, J. (1990). Sleep disturbances in child and adolescent psychiatric disorders. *Pediatrician*, **17**, 32–7.

Dahl, R. E., Ryan, N. D., Matty, M. K. et al. (1996). Sleep onset abnormalities in depressed adolescents. *Biological Psychiatry*, **39**, 400–10.

Dalla Bernardina, B., Colamaria, V., Chiamenti, C., Capovilla, G., Trevisan, E. & Tassinari, C. A. (1992). Benign partial epilepsy with affective symptoms (benign psychomotor epilepsy). In *Epileptic Syndromes in Infancy, Childhood and Adolescence*. 2nd edn, ed. J. Roger, M. Bureau, C. Dravet, F. E. Dreiffuss, A. Perret & P. Wolf, pp. 219–23. London: Libbey.

Dement, W. C. (1990). A personal history of sleep disorders medicine. *Journal of Clinical Neurophysiology*, **7**, 17–47.

Dement, W. C. & Mitler, M. M. (1993). It's time to wake up to the importance of sleep disorders. *Journal of the American Medical Association*, **269**, 1548–50.

Dickens, C. (1836/7). *The Posthumous Papers of the Pickwick Club*. London: Chapman & Hall. Published in serial form.

Dimario, F. J. & Emery, E. S. (1987). The natural history of night terrors. *Clinical Pediatrics*, **26**, 505–11.

Dinges, D. F. (1995). An overview of sleepiness and accidents. *Journal of Sleep Research*, **4**, supplement 2, 4–14.

Douglas, J. & Richman, N. (1984). *My Child Won't Sleep*. Harmondsworth: Penguin.

Douglass, A. B., Shipley, J. E., Haines, R. F., Scholten, R. C., Dudley, E. & Tapp, A. (1993). Schizophrenia, narcolepsy, and HLA-DR15, DQ6, *Biological Psychiatry*, **34**, 773–80.

Downey, R., Perkin, R. M. & MacQuarrie, J. (1993). Upper airway resistance syndrome: sick, symptomatic but unrecognized. *Sleep*, **16**, 620–3.

Dukes, C. (1905). Sleep in relation to education. *Journal of the Royal Sanitary Institute*, **26**, 41–4.

Education Committee of the General Medical Council (1993). *Tomorrow's Doctors. Recommendations on Undergraduate Medical Education*. London: General Medical Council.

Edwards, K. J. & Christopherson, E. R. (1994). Treating common sleep problems of young children. *Developmental and Behavioural Pediatrics*, **15**, 207–13.

Egger, J., Stolla, A. & McEwan, L. M. (1992). Controlled trial of hyposensitisation in children with food-induced hyperkinetic syndrome. *Lancet*, **339**, 1150–3.

Engleman, H. & Joffe, D. (1999). Neuropsychological function in obstructive sleep apnoea. *Sleep Medicine Reviews*, **3**, 59–78.

Ferber, R. (1986). *Solve Your Child's Sleep Problems*. London: Dorling Kindersley.

Ferber, R. (1987). Circadian and schedule disturbances. In *Sleep and its Disorders in Children*, ed. C. Guilleminault, pp. 165–75. New York: Raven Press.

Ferber, R. (1995). Circadian rhythm sleep disorders in childhood. In *Principles and Practice of*

Sleep Medicine in the Child, ed. R. Ferber & M. Kryger, pp. 91–8. Philadelphia: Saunders.

Ferber, R. & Boyle, M. D. (1983). Delayed sleep phase syndrome versus motivated sleep phase delay in adolescents. *Sleep Research*, **12**, 239.

Ferber, R. & Kryger, M. (eds.) (1995). *Principles and Practice of Sleep Medicine in the Child.* Philadelphia: Saunders.

Ficker, J. H., Wiest, G. H., Lehnert, G., Meyer, M. & Hahn, G. (1999). Are snoring medical students at risk of failing their exams? *Sleep*, **22**, 205–9.

Flint, J. (1996). Annotation: behavioural phenotypes: a window into the biology of behaviour. *Journal of Child Psychology and Psychiatry*, **37**, 355–67.

Ford, D. E. & Kamerow, D. B. (1989). Epidemiological study of sleep disturbances and psychiatric disorders: an opportunity for prevention? *Journal of the American Medical Association*, **262**, 1479–84.

France, K. G. & Hudson, S. M. (1990). Behaviour management of infant sleep disturbance. *Journal of Applied Behavior Analysis*, **23**, 91–8.

France, K. G. & Hudson, S. M. (1993). Management of infant sleep disturbance: a review. *Clinical Psychology Review*, **13**, 635–47.

France, K. G., Blampied, N. M. & Wilkinson, P. (1991). Treatment of infant sleep disturbance with trimeprazine in combination with behaviour management. *Journal of Developmental and Behavioral Pediatrics*, **12**, 308–14.

France, K. G., Henderson, J. M. T. & Hudson, M. (1996). Fact, act and tact. A three-stage approach to treating the sleep problems of infants and young children. *Child and Adolescent Psychiatric Clinics of North America*, **5**, 581–99.

Franck, L. S., Johnson, L. M., Lee, K. et al. (1999). Sleep disturbances in children with human immunodeficiency virus infection. *Pediatrics*, **104**, e62.

Frank, N. C., Spirito, A., Stark, L. & Owens-Stively, J. (1997). The use of scheduled awakenings to eliminate childhood sleepwalking. *Journal of Pediatric Psychology*, **22**, 345–53.

Fusco, L., Pachatz, C., Cusmai, R. & Vigevano, F. (1999). Repetitive sleep starts in neurologically impaired children: an unusual non-epileptic manifestation in otherwise epileptic subjects. *Epileptic Disorders*, **1**, 63–7.

Garland, E. J. (1995). The relationship of sleep disturbance to childhood panic disorder. In *Clinical Handbook of Sleep Disorders in Children*, ed. C. E. Shaefer, pp. 285–310. Northvale, NJ: Jason Aronson.

Garland, E. J. & Smith, D. H. (1991). Simultaneous prepubertal onset of panic disorder, night terrors, and somnambulism. *Journal of the American Academy of Child and Adolescent Psychiatry*, **30**, 553–5.

Gastaut, H. (1992). Benign epilepsy of childhood with occipital paroxysms. In *Epileptic Syndromes in Infancy, Childhood and Adolescence*, 2nd edn, ed. J. Roger, C. Dravet, M. Bureau, F. E. Dreiffus & P. Wolf, pp. 159–30. London: Libbey.

Gau, S. F. & Soong, W. T. (1999). Psychiatric comorbidity of adolescents with sleep terrors or sleepwalking: a case-control study. *Australian and New Zealand Journal of Psychiatry*, **33**, 734–9.

Gaultier, C. (1999). Sleep apnea in infants. *Sleep Medicine Reviews*, **3**, 303–12.

Geidd, J. N., Swedo, S. E., Lowe, C. H. & Rosenthal, N. E. (1998). Case series: seasonal affective disorder. A follow-up report. *Journal of the American Academy of Child and Adolescent Psychiatry*, **37**, 218–20.

Ghaem, M., Armstrong, K. L., Trocki, O., Cleghorn, G. J., Patrick, M. K. & Shepherd, R. W. (1998). The sleep patterns of infants and young children with gastro-oesophageal reflux. *Journal of Paediatrics and Child Health*, **34**, 160–3.

Gillberg, M. (1995). Sleepiness and its relation to the length, content and continuity of sleep. *Journal of Sleep Research*, **4**, supplement 2, 37–40.

Gillette, M. V., Roth, T. & Kiley, J. P. (1999). NIH funding of sleep research: a prospective and retrospective view. *Sleep*, **22**, 956–8.

Glod, C. A. & Baisden, N. (1999). Seasonal affective disorder in children and adolescents. *Journal of the American Psychiatric Nurses Association*, **5**, 29–33.

Glod, C. A., Teicher, M. H., Hartman, C. R. & Harakal, T. (1997). Increased nocturnal activity and impaired sleep maintenance in abused children. *Journal of the American Academy of Child and Adolescent Psychiatry*, **36**, 1236–43.

Golding, K. (1998). Nocturnal headbanging as a settling habit: the behavioural treatment of a 4 year old boy. *Clinical Child Psychology and Psychiatry*, **3**, 25–30.

Goodale, M. A. (1994). Active minds, sleeping bodies. *Lancet*, **344**, 1036–7.

Gormally, S. & Barr, R. G. (1997). Of clinical pies and clinical clues: proposal for a clinical approach to complaints of early crying and colic. *Ambulatory Child Health*, **3**, 137–53.

Gozal, D. (1998). Sleep disordered breathing and school performance in children. *Pediatrics*, **102**, 616–20.

Griffith, J. L. & Slovik, L. S. (1989). Munchausen syndrome by proxy and sleep disorders medicine. *Sleep*, **12**, 178–83.

Guilleminault, C. & Pelayo, R. (1998). Narcolepsy in prepubertal children. *Annals of Neurology*, **43**, 135–42.

Guilleminault, C. & Pelayo, R. (2000). Narcolepsy in children. A practical guide to its diagnosis, treatment and follow up. *Paediatric Drugs*, **2**, 1–9.

Guilleminault, C., Winkle, R., Korobkin, R. & Simmons, B. (1982). Children and nocturnal snoring: evaluation of the effects of sleep related resistive load and daytime functioning. *European Journal of Pediatrics*, **139**, 165–71.

Guilleminault, C., Pelayo, R., Leger, D., Clerk, A. & Bocian, R. C. Z. (1996). Recognition of sleep related breathing in children. *Pediatrics*, **98**, 871–82.

Hagerman, R. J., Riddle, J. E., Roberts, L. S., Breese, K. & Fulton, M. (1995). Survey of the efficacy of clonidine in fragile X syndrome. *Developmental Brain Dysfunction*, **8**, 336–44.

Harrison, Y. & Horne, J. A. (1995). Should we be taking more sleep? *Sleep*, **18**, 901–7.

Hewitt, K. & Galbraith, L. (1987). Postnatal classes on prevention of sleeplessness in young children. *Child: Care, Health and Development*, **13**, 415–20.

Hoeve, H. L., Joosten, K. F. & Van Den Berg, S. (1999). Management of obstructive sleep apnoea syndrome in children with craniofacial malformation. *International Journal of Pediatric Otorhinolaryngology*, **49**, supplement 1, 559–61.

Horne, J. A. (1988). Sleep loss and 'divergent' thinking ability. *Sleep*, **11**, 528–36.

Horne, J. A. (1991). Dimensions to sleepiness. In *Sleep, Sleepiness and Performance*, ed. T. H. Monk, pp. 169–95. Chichester: Wiley.

Horne, J. & Ostberg, O. (1979). Individual differences in human circadian rhythms. *Biological Psychology*, **5**, 179–90.

Hunt, A. & Stores, G. (1994). Sleep disorder and epilepsy in children with tuberous sclerosis: a questionnaire based study. *Developmental Medicine and Child Neurology*, **36**, 108–15.

Ishihara, K. (1999). The effect of 2-h sleep reduction by a delayed bedtime on daytime sleepiness in children. *Psychiatry and Clinical Neurosciences*, **53**, 113–15.

Jan, J. E., Espezel, H. & Appleton, R. E. (1994). The treatment of sleep disorders with melatonin. *Developmental Medicine and Child Neurology*, **36**, 97–107.

Jan, J. E., Connolly, M. B. C., Hamilton, D., Freeman, R. D. & Landon, M. (1999a). Melatonin treatment of non-epileptic myoclonus in children. *Developmental Medicine and Child Neurology*, **41**, 255–9.

Jan, J. E., Freeman, R. D. & Fast, D. K. (1999b). Melatonin treatment of sleep–wake cycle disorders in children and adolescents. *Developmental Medicine and Child Neurology*, **4**, 491–500.

Johns, M. (1998). Rethinking the assessment of sleepiness. *Sleep Medicine Reviews*, **2**, 3–15.

Johns, M. W. (2000). Sensitivity and specificity of the multiple sleep latency test (MSLT), the maintenance of wakefulness test and the Epworth sleepiness scale: Failure of the MSLT as a gold standard. *Journal of Sleep Research*, **9**, 5–11.

Kahn, A., Van de Merckt, C., Rebuffat, E. et al. (1989a). Sleep problems in healthy preadolescents. *Pediatrics*, **84**, 542–6.

Kahn, A., Mozin, M. J., Rebuffat, E., Sottiaux, M. & Muller, M. F. (1989b). Milk intolerance in children with persistent sleeplessness: a prospective double-blind crossover evaluation. *Pediatrics*, **84**, 595–603.

Kahn, A., Dan, B., Groswasser, J., Franco, P. & Sottiaux, M. (1996). Normal sleep architecture in infants and children. *Journal of Clinical Neurophysiology*, **13**, 184–97.

Kahn, Y. & Heckmatt, J. Z. (1996). Sleep in the healthy adolescent male. *Journal of Ambulatory Monitoring*, **9**, 355–64.

Kashden, J., Wise, M., Alvarado, I., Williams, M. & Boll, T. (1996). Neurocognitive functioning in children with narcolepsy. *Sleep Research*, **25**, 262.

Kavey, N. B. (1992). Psychosocial aspects of narcolepsy in children and adolescents. In *Psychosocial Aspects of Narcolepsy*, ed. M. Goswami, C. P. Pollak, F. L. Cohen, M. J. Thorpy & N. B. Kavey, pp. 91–101. New York: Haworth Press.

Kefauver, S. P. & Guilleminault, C. (1994). Sleep terrors and sleepwalking. In *Principles and Practice of Sleep Medicine,* 2nd edn, ed. M. H. Kryger, T. Roth & W. C. Dement, pp. 567–73. Philadelphia: Saunders.

Kennaway, D. J., Stamp, G. F. & Goble, F. C. (1992). Development of melatonin production in infants and the impact of prematurity. *Journal of Clinical Endocrinology and Metabolism*, **75**, 367–9.

Kerr, S. M., Jowett, S. A. & Smith, L. N. (1996). Preventing sleep problems in infants: a randomised control trial. *Journal of Advanced Nursing*, **24**, 938–42.

Kesler, A., Gadoth, N., Vainstein, G., Peled, R. & Lavie, P. (2000). Kleine Levin syndrome (KLS) in young females. *Sleep*, **23**, 563–7.

King, N., Ollendick, T. H. & Tonge, B. J. (1997). Children's nighttime fears. *Clinical Psychology Review*, **117**, 431–43.

Kirk, V., Kahn, A. & Brouillette, R. T. (1998). Diagnostic approach to obstructive sleep apnea in children. *Sleep Medicine Reviews*, **2**, 255–69.

Kirk, V. G., Morielli, A. & Brouillette, R. T. (1999). Sleep-disordered breathing in patients with myelomeningocele: the missed diagnosis. *Developmental Medicine and Child Neurology*, **41**, 40–3.

Koh, S., Ward, S. L., Lin, M. & Chen, L. S. (2000). Sleep apnea treatment improves seizure control in children with neurodevelopmental disorders. *Pediatric Neurology*, **22**, 36–9.

Kotagal, S., Gibbons, V. P. & Stith, J. A. (1994). Sleep abnormalities in patients with severe cerebral palsy. *Developmental Medicine and Child Neurology*, **36**, 304–11.

Kraemer, S. (2000). The fragile male. *British Medical Journal*, **321**, 1609–12.

Kramer, M., Schoen, L. S. & Kinney, L. (1984). The dream experiences in dreaming disturbed Vietnam veterans. In *Post-traumatic Stress Disorder: Psychological and Biological Sequelae*, ed. B. A. Van der Kolk, pp. 82–95. Washington: American Psychiatric Press.

Kravitz, M., McCoy, B. J., Tompkins, D. M. et al. (1993). Sleep disorders in children after burn injury. *Journal of Burn Care and Rehabilitation*, **14**, 83–90.

Kryger, M. H., Roth, T. & Dement, W. C. (2000). *Principles and Practice of Sleep Medicine*, 3rd edn. Philadelphia: Saunders.

Lancioni, G. E., O'Reilly, M. F. & Basili, G. (1999). Review of strategies for treating sleep problems in persons with severe or profound mental retardation or multiple handicaps. *American Journal of Mental Retardation*, **104**, 170–86.

Landry, P., Warnes, H., Nielson, T. & Montplaisir, J. (1999). Somnambulistic-like behaviour in patients attending a lithium clinic. *International Clinical Psychopharmacology*, **14**, 173–5.

Lavie, P. (1986). Ultrashort sleep-waking schedule III. 'Gates' and 'forbidden zones' for sleep. *Electroencephalography and Clinical Neurophysiology*, **63**, 414–25.

Lavie, P. (1993). Physician education in sleep disorders – a Dean of Medicine's viewpoint. *Sleep*, **16**, 760–1.

Lavigne, J. V., Arend, R., Rosenbaum, D. et al. (1999). Sleep and behavior problems among preschoolers. *Journal of Developmental and Behavioral Pediatrics*, **20**, 164–9.

Lawrence, J. W., Fauerbach, J., Endell, E., Ware, L. & Munster, A. (1998). The 1998 Clinical Research Award. Sleep disturbance after burn injury: a frequent yet understudied complication. *Journal of Burn Care and Rehabilitation*, **19**, 480–6.

Lawton, C., France, K. G. & Blampied, N. M. (1991). Treatment of infant sleep disturbance by graduated extinction. *Child and Family Behavior Therapy*, **13**, 39–56.

Leibenluft, J. (1999). The effects of caffeine on the sleep–wake cycles of children and adults. *Sleep Research Society Bulletin*, **5**, 50–1.

Levanon, A., Tarasiuk, A. & Tal, A. (1999). Sleep characteristics in children with Down syndrome. *Journal of Pediatrics*, **134**, 755–60.

Lewin, D. S. & Dahl, R. E. (1999). Importance of sleep in the management of pediatric pain. *Journal of Developmental and Behavioral Pediatrics*, **20**, 244–52.

Lillywhite, A. R., Wilson, S. J. & Nutt, D. J. (1994). Successful treatment of night terrors and somnambulism with paroxetine. *British Journal of Psychiatry*, **164**, 551–4.

Lindsley, J. G. (1992). Sleep paralysis. In *Movement Disorders in Neurology and Neuropsychiatry*, ed. A. B. Joseph & R. G. Young, pp. 602–19. Boston: Oxford University Press.

Loiseau, P. & Duché, B. (1989). Benign childhood epilepsy with centrotemporal spikes. *Cleveland Clinic Journal of Medicine*, **56**, supplement S17–S22.

Loughlin, G. M. & Carroll, J. L. (1995). Sleep and respiratory disease in children. In *Principles and Practice of Sleep Medicine in the Child*, ed. R. Ferber & M. Kryger, pp. 217–30. Philadelphia: Saunders.

Loughlin, G. M., Brouillette, R. T., Brooke, L. J. et al. (1996). American Thoracic Society standards and indications for cardiopulmonary sleep studies in children. *American Journal of Respiratory and Critical Care Medicine*, **153**, 866–78.

Lozoff, B. (1995). Culture and family: influences on childhood sleep practices and problems. In *Principles and Practice of Sleep Medicine in the Child*, ed. R. Ferber & M. Kryger, pp. 69–73. Philadelphia: Saunders.

Macknin, M. L., Piedmonte, M., Jacobs, J. & Skibinski, C. (2000). Symptoms associated with infant teething: a prospective study. *Pediatrics*, **105**, 747–52.

McArthur, A. J. & Budden, S. S. (1998). Sleep dysfunction in Rett syndrome: a trial of exogenous melatonin treatment. *Developmental Medicine and Child Neurology*, **40**, 186–92.

McClellan, K. J. & Spencer, C. M. (1998). Modafinil. A review of its pharmacology and clinical efficacy in the management of narcolepsy. *CNS Drugs*, **9**, 311–24.

McColley, S. A., Carroll, J. L., Curtis, S., Loughlin, G. M. & Sampson, H. A. (1997). High prevalence of allergic sensitization in children with habitual snoring and obstructive sleep apnea. *Chest*, **111**, 170–3.

McGraw, K., Hoffman, R., Harker, C. & Herman, J. H. (1999). The development of circadian rhythms in a human infant. *Sleep*, **22**, 303–10.

Mahowald, M. W. & Schenck, C. H. (1992). Dissociated states of wakefulness and sleep. *Neurology*, **42**, supplement 6, 44–52.

Mahowald, M. W. & Schenck, C. H. (1996). NREM sleep parasomnias. *Neurologic Clinics*, **14**, 675–96.

Mahowald, M. W. & Schenck, C. H. (2000). REM sleep parasomnias. In *Principles and Practice of Sleep Medicine*, 3rd edn, ed. M. H. Kryger, T. Roth & W. C. Dement, pp. 724–41. Philadelphia: Saunders.

Malow, B. A., Bowes, R. J. & Lin, X. (1997). Predictors of sleepiness in epilepsy patients. *Sleep*, **20**, 1105–10.

Manners, P. (1999). Are growing pains a myth? *Australian Family Physician*, **28**, 124–7.

Maquet, R. (1999). Brain mechanisms of sleep: contribution of neuroimaging techniques. *Journal of Psychopharmacology*, **13**, supplement 1, S25–8.

Marcus, C. L. (2000). Obstructive sleep apnea: differences between children and adults. *Sleep*, **23**, S140–S141.

Marcus, C. L., Omlin, K. J., Basinski, D. J. et al. (1992). Normal polysomnographic values for children and adolescents. *American Review of Respiratory Disease*, **146**, 1235–9.

Matyka, K., Crawford, C., Wiggs, L., Dunger, D. B. & Stores, G. (2000). Alterations in sleep physiology in young children with insulin dependant diabetes mellitus: relationships to nocturnal hypoglycaemia. *Journal of Pediatrics*, 137, 233–8.

Maurer, K. E. & Schaefer, C. E. (1998). Assessment and treatment of children's nightmares: a review. *Psychology: a Journal of Human Behaviour*, **35**, 30–6.

Meijer, A. M., Habekothé, H. T. & Van Den Wittenboer, G. L. H. (2000). Time in bed, quality of sleep and school functioning of children. *Journal of Sleep Research*, **9**, 145–53.

Mendelson, W. B. (1994). Sleepwalking associated with zolpidem. *Journal of Clinical Psychopharmacology*, **14**, 150.

Mignot, E. (2000). Perspectives in narcolepsy and hypocretin (orexin) research (editorial). *Sleep Medicine*, **1**, 87–90.

Minde, K., Faucon, A. & Falkner, S. (1994). Sleep problems in toddlers, effects of treatment on their daytime behavior. *Journal of the American Academy of Child and Adolescent Psychiatry*, **33**, 1114–21.

Mindell, J. A. (1993). Sleep disorders in children. *Health Psychology*, **12**, 151–62.

Mindell, J. A. (1999). Empirically supported treatments in pediatric psychology: bedtime refusal and night wakings in young children. *Journal of Pediatric Psychology*, **24**, 465–81.

Mindell, J. A., Owens, J. A. & Carskadon, M. A. (1999). Developmental features of sleep. *Child and Adolescent Psychiatric Clinics of North America*, **8**, 695–725.

Miser, A. W., McCalla, J., Dothage, J. A., Wesley, M. & Miser, J. A. (1987). Pain as a presenting symptom in children and young adults with newly diagnosed malignancy. *Pain*, **29**, 85–90.

Mitler, M. M. (1996). Sleepiness and human behaviour. *Current Opinion in Pulmonary Medicine*, **2**, 488–91.

Mitler, M., Aldrich, M. S., Koob, G. F. & Zarcone, V. P. (1994). Narcolepsy and its treatment with stimulants. *Sleep*, **17**, 352–71.

Mitler, M. M. & Miller, J. C. (1996). Methods of testing for sleepiness. *Behavioral Medicine*, **21**, 171–83.

Moffat, M. E. K. (1997). Nocturnal enuresis: a review of the efficacy of treatments and practical advice for clinicians. *Developmental and Behavioral Pediatrics*, **18**, 49–56.

Molaie, M. & Deutsch, G. K. (1997). Psychogenic events presenting as parasomnia. *Sleep*, **20**, 402–5.

Moldofsky, H. & Dickstein, J. B. (1999). Sleep and cytokine-immune functions in medical, psychiatric and primary sleep disorders. *Sleep Medicine Reviews*, **3**, 325–37.

Moline, M. L. & Zendell, S. M. (1993). Sleep education in professional training programs. *Sleep Research*, **22**, 1.

Montagna, P. (2000). Motor disorders of sleep. In *Sleep Disorders and Neurological Disease*, ed. A. Culebras, pp. 193–215. New York: Marcel Dekker.

Montgomery, P. & Stores, G. (2000). Behavioural treatment of sleep disorders in children with learning disability (mental retardation): a randomised controlled trial of treatment delivery methods. *Journal of Sleep Research*, **9**, supplement 1, S135.

Montplaisir, J., Michaud, M., Denesle, R. & Gosselin, A. (2000). Periodic leg movements are not more prevalent in insomnia or hypersomnia but are specifically associated with sleep disorders involving a dopaminergic impairment. *Sleep Medicine*, **1**, 163–7.

Morrell, J. M. B. (1999). The role of maternal cognitions in infant sleep disorder as assessed by a new instrument, the Maternal Cognitions Questionnaire. *Journal of Child Psychology and Psychiatry*, **40**, 247–58.

Morrison, D. N., McGee, R. & Stanton, W. R. (1992). Sleep problems in adolescence. *Journal of the American Academy of Child and Adolescent Psychiatry*, **31**, 94–9.

Muris, P., Merckelbach, H., Gadet, B. & Moulaert, V. (2000). Fears, worries and scary dreams in 4 to 12 year old children: their content, developmental pattern, and origins. *Journal of Clinical Child Psychology*, **29**, 43–52.

National Commission on Sleep Disorders Research. (1993). *Wake Up America: A National Sleep Alert*. Vol. 1, *Executive Summary and Report*. Bethesda, MD: Department of Health and Human Sciences.

National Commission on Sleep Disorders Research. (1994). *Wake Up America: A National Sleep Alert*. Vol. 2, *Working Group Reports*. Bethesda, MD: Department of Health and Human Sciences.

Naylor, M. W. & Aldrich, M. S. (1991). The distribution of confusional arousals across sleep stages and time of night in children and adolescents with sleep terrors. *Sleep Research*, **20**, 308.

Obermeyer, W. H. & Benca, R. M. (1996). Effects of drugs on sleep. *Neurologic Clinics*, **14**, 827–40.

O'Callaghan, F. J. K., Clarke, A. A., Hancock, E., Hunt, A. & Osborne, J. P. (1999). Use of melatonin to treat sleep disorders in tuberous sclerosis. *Developmental Medicine and Child Neurology*, **41**, 123–6.

Ohayon, M. M., Guilleminault, C. & Priest, R. G. (1999). Night terrors, sleep walking, and confusional arousals in the general population: their frequency and relationship to other sleep and mental disorders. *Journal of Clinical Psychiatry*, **60**, 268–76.

Oishibashi, Y., Kakizawa, T., Otsuka, A. et al. (1993). Disturbances of sleep waking in handicapped children (II): trend of circadian rhythm disorders in deaf children. *Japanese Journal of Psychiatry and Neurology*, **47**, 464–5.

Oldani, A., Zucconi, M., Castronovo, C. & Ferini-Strambi, L. (1998). Nocturnal frontal lobe epilepsy misdiagnosed as sleep apnoea syndrome. *Acta Neurologica Scandinavica*, **98**, 67–71.

Osler, W. (1982). Chronic tonsillitis. In *Principles and Practice of Medicine*, pp. 335–9. New York: Appleton.

Oswald, I. & Evans, J. (1985). On serious violence during sleepwalking. *British Journal of Psychiatry*, **149**, 120–1.

Owens, J., Opipari, L., Nobile, C. & Spirito, A. (1998). Sleep and daytime behavior in children with obstructive sleep apnea and behavioral sleep disorders. *Pediatrics*, **102**, 1178–84.

Owens, J. L., France, K. G. & Wiggs, L. (1999a). Behavioural and cognitive-behavioural interventions for sleep disorders in infants and children: a review. *Sleep Medicine Reviews*, **3**, 281–302.

Owens, J., Maxim, R., McGuinn, M., Nobile, C., Msall, M. & Alario, A. (1999b). Television-viewing habits and sleep disturbance in school children. *Pediatrics*, **104**, e27.

Owens, J. A., Spirito, A., McGuinn, M. & Nobile, C. (2000). Sleep habits and sleep disturbance in elementary school-age children. *Developmental and Behavioral Pediatrics*, **21**, 27–36.

Owens-Stively, J., Spirito, A. & Arrigan, M. (1996). The incidence of parasomnias in children with obstructive sleep apnea. *Sleep*, **20**, 1193–6.

Palace, E. M. & Johnston, C. (1989). Treatment of recurrent nightmares by the dream re-organisation approach. *Journal of Behaviour Therapy and Experimental Psychiatry*, **20**, 219–26.

Palm, E., Personn, D., Elmqvist, D. & Blennow, G. (1989). Sleep and wakefulness in normal preadolescent children. *Sleep*, **12**, 299–328.

Panayiotopolous, C. P. (1999). Early-onset benign childhood occipital seizure susceptibility syndrome: a syndrome to recognize. *Epilepsia*, **40**, 621–30.

Parkes, D. J. (1999). Genetic factors in human sleep disorders with special reference to Norrie disease, Prader–Willi syndrome and Moebius syndrome. *Journal of Sleep Research*, **8**, supplement 1, 14–22.

Parkes, J. D., Chen, S. Y., Clift, S. J., Dahlitz, M. J. & Dunn, G. (1998). The clinical diagnosis of the narcoleptic syndrome. *Journal of Sleep Research*, **7**, 41–52.

Patzold, L. M., Richdale, A. L. & Tongue, B. J. (1998). An investigation into sleep characteristics of children with autism and Asperger's syndrome. *Journal of Paediatrics and Child Health*, **34**, 528–33.

Perrin, S., Smith, P. & Yule, W. (2000). Practitioner review: the assessment and treatment of post-traumatic stress disorder in children and adolescents. *Journal of Child Psychology and Psychiatry*, **41**, 277–89.

Phaire, T. (1545). *The Boke of Chyldren*. Translation by A. V. Neale and H. R. E. Wallis. Edinburgh: Livingstone, 1955.

Philip, P. & Guilleminault, C. (1996). Adult psychophysiological insomnia and positive history of childhood insomnia. *Sleep*, **19**, 516–22.

Phillips, K. D. (1999). Physiological and pharmacological factors of insomnia in HIV disease. *Journal of the Association of Nurses in AIDS Care*, **10**, 93–7.

Piazza, C. C., Fisher, W. W. & Acherer, M. (1997). Treatment of multiple sleep problems in children with developmental difficulties: faded bedtime with response cost versus bedtime scheduling. *Developmental Medicine and Child Neurology*, **39**, 414–18.

Picchietti, D. L. & Walters, A. S. (1999). Moderate to severe periodic limb movement disorder in childhood and adolescence. *Sleep*, **22**, 297–300.

Picchietti, D. L., Underwood, D. J., Farris, W. A. et al. (1999). Further studies on periodic limb movement disorder and restless legs syndrome in children with attention-deficit hyperactivity disorder. *Movement Disorders*, **14**, 1000–7.

Pike, M. & Stores, G. (1994). Kleine–Levin syndrome: a cause of diagnostic confusion. *Archives of Disease in Childhood*, **71**, 355–7.

Pilcher, J. J. & Huffcutt, A. I. (1996). Effects of sleep deprivation on performance: a meta-analysis. *Sleep*, **19**, 318–26.

Pinchbeck, I. & Hewitt, M. (1969). *Children in English Society Vol. 1. From Tudor Times to the Eighteenth Century*. London: Routledge and Kegan Paul.

Pollock, J. I. (1994). Nightwaking at five years of age: predictors and prognosis. *Journal of Clinical Psychology and Psychiatry*, **35**, 699–708.

Popper, C. W. (1995). Combining methylphenidate with clonidine: Pharmacologic questions and news reports about sudden death. *Journal of Child and Adolescent Psychopharmacology*, **5**, 157–66.

Prince, J. B., Wilens, T. E., Biederman, J., Spencer, T. J. & Wozniak, J. R. (1996). Clonidine for sleep disturbances associated with attention-deficit hyperactivity disorder: a systematic chart review of 62 cases. *Journal of the American Academy of Child and Adolescent Psychiatry*, **35**, 599–605.

Pritchard, A. & Appleton, P. (1988). Management of sleep problems in pre-school children. *Early Child Development and Care*, **34**, 227–40.

Provini, F., Plazzi, G., Tinuper, P., Vandi, S., Lugaresi, G. & Montagna, P. (1999). Nocturnal frontal lobe epilepsy. A clinical and polygraphic review of 100 consecutive cases. *Brain*, **122**, 1017–31.

Quine, L. (1992). Severity of sleep problems in children with severe learning difficulties: description and correlates. *Journal of Community and Applied Social Psychology*, **2**, 247–68.

Quine, L. (1997). *Solving Children's Sleep Problems*. Huntingdon: Beckett Karlson.

Ramchandani, P., Wiggs, L., Webb, V. & Stores, G. (2000). A systematic review of treatments for settling and night waking problems in children. *British Medical Journal*, **320**, 209–13.

Randazzo, A. C., Muchlebach, M. J., Schweitzer, P. K. & Walsh, J. K. (1998). Cognitive function following acute sleep restriction in children ages 10–14. *Sleep*, **21**, 861–8.

Rechtschaffen, A. (1998). Current perspectives on the function of sleep. *Perspectives in Biology and Medicine*, **41**, 359–90.

Rechtschaffen, A. & Kales, A. (1968). *A Manual of Standardised Terminology, Techniques and Scoring System for Sleep Stages of Human Subjects*. UCLA Brain Information Service, Brain Research Institute, Los Angeles CA.

Regestein, Q. R. & Monk, T. H. (1995). Delayed sleep phase syndrome: a review of its clinical aspects. *American Journal of Psychiatry*, **152**, 602–8.

Reynolds, C. F. (1989). Sleep disturbance in posttraumatic stress disorder: pathogenetic or epiphenomenal? *American Journal of Psychiatry*, **146**, 695–6.

Richdale, A. L., Cotton, S. & Hibbit, K. (1999). Sleep and behaviour disturbance in Prader–Willi syndrome: a questionnaire study. *Journal of Intellectual Disability Research*, **43**, 380–92.

Richman, N. (1987). Surveys of sleep disorders in children in a general population. In *Sleep and its Disorders in Children*, ed. C. Guilleminault, pp. 115–27. New York: Raven Press.

Rickert, V. I. & Johnson, C. M. (1998). Reducing nocturnal awakening and crying episodes in infants and young children: a comparison between scheduled awakenings and systematic ignoring. *Pediatrics*, **81**, 203–12.

Rizzardo, R., Savastano, M., Maron, M. B., Mangialaio, M. & Salvadori, L. (1998). Psychological distress in patients with tinnitus. *Journal of Otolaryngology*, **27**, 21–5.

Roberts, C. & Hindley, P. (1999). Practitioner review: the assessment and treatment of deaf children with psychiatric disorders. *Journal of Child Psychology and Psychiatry*, **40**, 151–67.

Roberts, R. N. & Gordon, S. B. (1979). Reducing childhood nightmares subsequent to burn trauma. *Child Behaviour Therapy*, **1**, 373–81.

Rona, R. J., Li, L. & Chin, S. (1997). Determinants of nocturnal enuresis in England and Scotland in the '90s. *Developmental Medicine and Child Neurology*, **39**, 677–81.

Rosen, C. L., D'Andrea, L. & Haddad, G. G. (1992). Adult criteria for obstructive sleep apnea do not identify children with serious obstruction. *American Review of Respiratory Disease*, **146**, 1231–4.

Rosen, G., Mahowald, M. W. & Ferber, R. (1995). Sleepwalking, confusional arousals, and sleep terrors in the child. In *Principles and Practice of Sleep Medicine in the Child*, ed. R. Ferber & M. Kryger, pp. 99–106. Philadelphia: Saunders.

Rosen, J., Blennow, G., Risberg, A. M. & Ingvar, D. H. (1982). Quantitative evaluation of nocturnal sleep in epileptic children. In *Sleep and Epilepsy*, ed. M. B. Sterman, M. N. Shouse & P. Passonant, pp. 397–409. New York: Academic Press.

Rosen, R. C., Rosekind, M., Rosevaar, C., Cole, W. E. & Dement, W. C. (1993). Physician education in sleep and sleep disorders: a national survey of US medical schools. *Sleep*, **16**, 249–54.

Roth, T., Roehrs, T. A., Carskadon, M. A. & Dement, W. C. (1994). Daytime sleepiness and alertness. In *Principles and Practice of Sleep Medicine*, 2nd edn, ed. M. H. Kryger, T. Roth & W. C. Dement, pp. 40–9. Philadelphia: Saunders.

Royal College of Paediatrics and Child Health (1996). *Syllabus and Training Record for General Professional and Higher Specialist Training in Paediatrics and Child Health*. London: Royal College of Paediatrics and Child Health.

Ryan, N. D., Puig-Antich, J., Rabinovich, H. et al. (1987). The clinical picture of major depression in children and adolescents. *Archives of General Psychiatry*, **44**, 854–61.

Rye, D. B., Johnston, L. H., Watts, R. L. & Bliwise, D. L. (1999). Juvenile Parkinson's disease with REM sleep behavior disorder, sleepiness and daytime REM onset. *Neurology*, **53**, 1868–70.

Sachs, C. & Svanborg, E. (1991). The exploding head syndrome: polysomnographic recordings and therapeutic suggestions. *Sleep*, **14**, 263–6.

Sadeh, A. (1994). Assessment of intervention for infant night waking: parental reports and activity-based monitoring. *Journal of Consulting and Clinical Psychology*, **62**, 63–8.

Sadeh, A. (1996). Stress, trauma, and sleep in children. *Child and Adolescent Psychiatric Clinics of North America*, **6**, 685–700.

Sadeh, A. & Anders, T. F. (1993). Infant sleep problems: origins, assessment, intervention. *Infant Mental Health Journal*, **14**, 1–34.

Sadeh, A,, Levie, P., Scher, A., Tirosh, E. & Epstein, R. (1991). Actigraphic home-monitoring sleep-disturbed and control infants and young children: a new method for pediatric assessment of sleep–wake patterns. *Pediatrics*, **87**, 494–9.

Sadeh, A., McGuire, J. P. D., Sachs, H. et al. (1995). Sleep and psychological characteristics of children on a psychiatric inpatient unit. *Journal of the American Academy of Child Adolescent and Psychiatry*, **34**, 813–19.

Sadeh, A., Horowitz, I., Wolach-Benodis, L. & Wolach, B. (1998). Sleep and pulmonary function in children with well-controlled stable asthma. *Sleep*, **21**, 379–84.

Sadeh, A., Raviv, A. & Gruber, R. (2000). Sleep patterns and sleep disruption in school-age children. *Developmental Psychology*, **36**, 291–301.

Sadler, M. (1999). Lamotrigine associated with insomnia. *Epilepsia*, **40**, 322–5.

Salinsky, M. C., Oken, B. S. & Binder, L. M. (1996). Assessment of drowsiness in epilepsy patients receiving chronic antiepileptic drug therapy. *Epilepsia*, **37**, 181–7.

Salzarulo, P. (1990). Workshop on education about sleep in Europe: chairman's summary. In *Sleep '90. Proceedings of the Tenth European Congress on Sleep Research*, ed. J. A. Horne, pp. 475–8. Bochum: Pontnagel Press.

Salzarulo, P. & Chevalier, A. (1983). Sleep problems in children and their relationships with early disturbances of the waking–sleeping rhythms. *Sleep*, **6**, 47–51.

Samuels, M. P., Stebbens, V. A., Davies, S. C., Picton-Jones, E. & Southall, D. P. (1992). Sleep related upper airway obstruction and hypoxaemia in sickle cell disease. *Archives of Disease in Childhood*, **67**, 925–9.

Scheffer, I. E., Bhatia, K. P., Lopes-Cendes, I. et al. (1995). Autosomal dominant nocturnal frontal lobe epilepsy. A distinctive clinical disorder. *Brain*, **118**, 61–73.

Schenck, C. H. & Mahowald, M. W. (1996). Long-term, nightly benzodiazepine treatment of injurious parasomnias and other disorders of disrupted sleep in 170 adults. *American Journal of Medicine*, **100**, 333–7.

Schenck, C. H., Milner, D. M., Hurwitz, T. D., Bundlie, S. R. & Mahowald, M. W. (1989). Dissociative disorders presenting as somnambulism: polysomnographic, video and clinical documentation (8 cases). *Dissociation*, **2**, 194–204.

Schenck, C. H., Hurwitz, T. D., O'Connor, K. A. & Mahowald, M. W. (1993). Additional categories of sleep-related eating disorders and the current status of treatment. *Sleep*, **16**, 457–66.

Schenck, C. H., Boyd, J. L. & Mahowald, M. W. (1997). A parasomnia overlap disorder involving sleepwalking, sleep terrors, and REM sleep behavior disorder in 33 polysomnographically confirmed cases. *Sleep*, **20**, 972–81.

Scott, G. & Richards, M. P. M. (1990). Night waking in infants: effects of providing advice and support for parents. *Journal of Child Psychology and Psychiatry*, **31**, 551–67.

Seifer, R., Sameroff, A. J., Dickstein, S., Hayden, L. C. & Schiller, M. (1996). Parental psychopathology and sleep variation in children. *Child and Adolescent Psychiatric Clinics of North America*, **5**, 715–27.

Sforza, E., Krieger, J. & Petiau, C. (1997). REM sleep behavior disorder: clinical and physiopathological findings. *Sleep Medicine Reviews*, **1**, 57–69.

Sheldon, S. H., Ahart, S. & Levy, H. B. (1991). Sleep patterns in abused and neglected children. *Sleep Research*, **20**, 333.

Sheldon, S. H. & Jacobsen, J. (1998). REM-sleep motor disorder in children. *Journal of Child Neurology*, **13**, 257–60.

Sheldon, S. H., Spire, J.-P. & Levy, H. B. (1992). Sleep wake schedule disorders. In *Pediatric Sleep Medicine*, ed. S. H. Sheldon, J.-P. Spire & H. B. Levy, pp. 106–18. Philadelphia: Saunders.

Silverman, M. (1988). Airway obstruction and sleep disruption in Down's syndrome. *British Medical Journal*, **296**, 1618–19.

Simonds, J. F. & Parraga, H. (1982). Prevalence of sleep disorders and sleep behaviors in children and adolescents. *Journal of the American Academy of Child Psychiatry*, **21**, 383–8.

Simonds, J. F. & Parraga, H. (1984). Sleep behaviors and disorders in children and adolescents evaluated at psychiatric clinics. *Developmental and Behavioral Pediatrics*, **5**, 6–10.

Soriani, S., Carrozzi, M., DeCarlo, L. et al. (1997). Endozepine stupor in children. *Cephalalgia*, **17**, 658–61.

Steiger, A. & Holsboer, F. (1997). Neuropeptides and human sleep. *Sleep*, **20**, 1038–52.

Stein, M. A. (1999). Unravelling sleep problems in treated and untreated children with ADHD. *Journal of Child and Adolescent Psychopharmacology*, **9**, 157–68.

St James-Roberts, I. (1992). Managing infants who cry persistently. *British Medical Journal*, **304**, 997–8.

St James-Roberts, I., Conroy, S. & Wilsher, K. (1996). Bases for maternal perceptions of infant crying and colic behaviour. *Archives of Disease in Childhood*, **75**, 375–84.

Stoléru, S., Nottelmann, E. D., Belmont, B. & Ronsaville, D. (1997). Sleep problems in children of affectively ill mothers. *Journal of Child Psychology and Psychiatry*, **38**, 831–41.

Stores, G. (1985). Clinical and EEG evaluation of seizures and seizure-like disorders. *Journal of the American Academy of Child Psychiatry*, **24**, 10–16.

Stores, G. (1991). Confusions concerning sleep disorders and the epilepsies in children and adolescents. *British Journal of Psychiatry*, **158**, 1–7.

Stores, G. (1992). Annotation: sleep studies in children with a mental handicap. *Journal of Child Psychology and Psychiatry*, **33**, 1303–17.

Stores, G. (1994). Investigation of sleep disorders including home monitoring. *Archives of Disease in Childhood*, **71**, 184–5.

Stores, G. (1996). Practitioner review: assessment and treatment of sleep disorders in children and adolescents. *Journal of Child Psychology and Psychiatry*, **37**, 907–25.

Stores, G. (1998). Sleep paralysis and hallucinosis. *Behavioural Neurology*, **11**, 109–12.

Stores, G. (1999a). Recognition and management of narcolepsy. *Archives of Disease in Childhood*, **81**, 519–24.

Stores, G. (1999b). Sleep disturbance in chronic fatigue syndrome. *Association for Child Psychology and Psychiatry Occasional Papers*, No. 16, 13–17.

Stores, G. & Crawford, C. (1998). Medical student education in sleep and its disorders. *Journal of the Royal College of Physicians of London*, **32**, 149–53.

Stores, G. & Crawford, C. (2000). Arousal norms for children age 5–16 years based on home polysomnography. *Technology and Health Care*, **8**, 259–64.

Stores, G. & Ramchandani, P. (1999). Sleep disorders in visually impaired children. *Developmental Medicine and Child Neurology*, **41**, 348–52.

Stores, G. & Wiggs, L. (1998a). Abnormal sleep patterns associated with autism and related syndromes. *Autism*, **2**, 157–69.

Stores, G. & Wiggs, L. (1998b). Clinical services for sleep disorders. *Archives of Disease in Childhood*, **79**, 495–7.

Stores, G. & Wiggs, L. (2001). *Sleep Disturbance in Disorders of Development: its Significance and Management*. London: Mac Keith Press.

Stores, G., Zaiwalla, Z. & Bergel, N. (1991). Frontal lobe complex partial seizures in children: a form of epilepsy at particular risk of misdiagnosis. *Developmental Medicine and Child Neurology*, **33**, 998–1009.

Stores, G., Zaiwalla, Z., Styles, E. & Hoshika, A. (1995). Nonconvulsive status epilepticus. *Archives of Disease in Childhood*, **73**, 106–11.

Stores, G., Crawford, C., Selman, J. & Wiggs, L. (1998a). Home polysomnography norms for children. *Technology and Health Care*, **6**, 231–6.

Stores, G., Fry, A. & Crawford, C. (1998b). Sleep abnormalities demonstrated by home polysomnography in teenagers with the chronic fatigue syndrome. *Journal of Psychosomatic Research*, **45**, 85–92.

Stores, G., Ellis, A. J., Wiggs, L., Crawford, C. & Thomson, A. (1998c). Sleep and psychological disturbance in nocturnal asthma. *Archives of Disease in Childhood*, **78**, 413–19.

Stores, G., Burrows, A. & Crawford, C. (1998d). Physiological sleep disturbance in children with atopic dermatitis: a case control study. *Pediatric Dermatology*, **15**, 264–8.

Stores, G., Wiggs, L. & Campling, G. (1998e). Sleep disorders and their relation to psychological disturbance in children with epilepsy. *Child: Care, Health and Development*, **24**, 5–19.

Stores, R. & Wiggs, L. (1998). Sleep education in clinical psychology courses in the UK. *Clinical Psychology Forum*, **119**, 14–18.

Stores, R., Stores, G. & Buckley, S. (1996). The pattern of sleep problems in children with Down's syndrome and other intellectual disabilities. *Journal of Applied Research in Intellectual Disabilities*, **9**, 145–59.

Stores, R., Stores, G., Fellows, B. & Buckley, S. (1998). A factor analysis of sleep problems and their psychological associations in children with Down's syndrome. *Journal of Applied Research in Intellectual Disabilities*, **11**, 345–54.

Swedo, S. E., Allen, A. J., Glod, C. A. et al. (1997). A controlled trial of light therapy for the treatment of pediatric seasonal affective disorder. *Journal of the American Academy of Child and Adolescent Psychiatry*, **36**, 816–21.

Sweitzer, P. K. (2000). Drugs that disturb sleep and wakefulness. In *Principles and Practice of Sleep Medicine*, 3rd edn, ed. M. H. Kryger, T. Roth & W. C. Derment, pp. 441–61. Philadelphia: Saunders.

Sykes, G. (1999). The role of sleep clinics in helping children get a good night's rest. *Community Nurse*, supplement **5**, S13–S14.

Szymczak, J. T., Jasinska, M., Pawlak, E. & Zweirzykowska, M. (1993). Annual and weekly changes in the sleep–wake rhythms of school children. *Sleep*, **16**, 433–5.

Tachibana, N., Kimura, K., Kitajima, K., Shinde, A., Kimura, J. & Shibasaki, H. (1997). REM sleep motor dysfunction in multiple system atrophy: with special emphasis on sleep talk as its early clinical manifestation. *Journal of Neurology, Neurosurgery and Psychiatry*, **63**, 678–81.

Tasker, R. C., Dundas, I., Laverty, A., Fletcher, M., Lane, R. & Stocks, J. (1998). Distinct patterns of respiratory difficulty in young children with achondroplasia: a clinical, sleep and lung function study. *Archives of Disease in Childhood*, **79**, 99–108.

Tassinari, C. A., Mancia, D., Dalla Bernadina, B. & Gastaut, H. (1972). Pavor nocturnus of nonepileptic nature in epileptic children. *Electroencephalography and Clinical Neurophysiology*, **33**, 603–7.

Taylor, B. J. & Brooks, C. G. D. (1986). Sleep EEG in growth disorders. *Archives of Disease in Childhood*, **61**, 754–60.

Terzano, M. G. & Parrino, L. (2000). Origin and significance of the cyclic alternating pattern (CAP). *Sleep Medicine Reviews*, **4**, 101–23.

Thacker, K., Devinsky, O., Perrine, K., Alper, K. & Luciano, D. (1993). Nonepileptic seizures during apparent sleep. *Annals of Neurology*, **33**, 414–18.

Thorpy, M. J. (1990a). Rhythmic movement disorder. In *Handbook of Sleep Disorders*, ed. M. J. Thorpy, pp. 609–29. New York: Marcel Dekker.

Thorpy, M. J. (1990b). Disorders of arousal. In *Handbook of Sleep Disorders*, ed. M. J. Thorpy, pp. 531–49. New York: Marcel Dekker.

Thorpy, M. J. (2000). Historical perspective on sleep and man. In *Sleep Disorders and Neurological Disease*, ed. A. Culebras, pp. 1–36. Marcel Dekker: New York.

Thorpy, M. J., Korman, E., Spielman, A. J. & Glorinsky, P. B. (1988). Delayed sleep phase syndrome in adolescents. *Journal of Adolescent Health Care*, **9**, 22–7.

Tinuper, P., Cerullo, A., Cirignotta, F., Cortelli, P., Lugaresi, F. & Montagna, P. (1990). Nocturnal paroxysmal dystonia with short-lasting attacks: three cases with evidence for an epileptic origin of seizures. *Epilepsia*, **3**, 549–56.

Tirosh, E. & Borochowitz, Z. (1992). Sleep apnea in fragile X syndrome. *American Journal of Medical Genetics*, **43**, 124–7.

Trenkwalder, C., Walters, A. S. & Hening, W. (1996). Periodic limb movements and restless legs syndrome. *Neurologic Clinics*, **14**, 629–50.

Tynjälä, J., Kannas, L. & Välimaa, R. (1993). How young Europeans sleep. *Health Education Research Theory and Practice*, **8**, 69–80.

Tynjälä, J., Kannas, L. & Levälahti, E. (1997). Perceived tiredness among adolescents and its association with sleep habits and use of psychoactive substances. *Journal of Sleep Research*, **6**, 189–98.

Udwin, O., Yule, W. & Martin, N. (1987). Cognitive abilities and behavioural characteristics of children with idiopathic infantile hypercalcaemia. *Journal of Child Psychology and Psychiatry*, **28**, 297–309.

Waldhauser, F., Weisenbacher, G., Tatzer, E. et al. (1988). Alterations in nocturnal serum melatonin levels in humans with growth and ageing. *Journal of Clinical Endocrinology and Metabolism*, **66**, 648–52.

Weissbluth, M. (1995a). Naps in children: 6 months to 7 years. *Sleep*, **18**, 82–7.

Weissbluth, M. (1995b). Colic. In *Principles and Practice of Sleep Medicine in the Child*, ed. R. Ferber & M. Kryger, pp. 75–8. Philadelphia: Saunders.

White, M. A., Williams, P. D., Alexander, D. J., Powell-Cope, G. M. & Conlon, M. (1990). Sleep onset latency and distress in hospitalised children. *Nursing Research*, **39**, 134–9.

Wiggs, L. & France, K. (2000). Behavioural treatments for sleep problems in children and adolescents with physical illness, psychological problems or intellectual disabilities. *Sleep Medicine Reviews*, **4**, 299–314.

Wiggs, L. & Stores, G. (1995). Children's sleep: how should it be assessed? *Association of Child Psychology and Psychiatry Review and Newsletter*, **17**, 153–7.

Wiggs, L. & Stores, G. (1996). Sleep problems in children with severe intellectual disabilities: what help is being provided? *Journal of Applied Research in Intellectual Disabilities*, **9**, 160–5.

Wiggs, L. & Stores, G. (1998). Behavioural treatment for sleep problems in children with severe learning disabilities and daytime challenging behaviour: effect on sleep patterns of mother and child. *Journal of Sleep Research*, **7**, 119–26.

Wiggs, L. & Stores, R. (1996). Sleep education in undergraduate psychology degree courses in the UK. *Psychology Teaching Review*, **5**, 40–6.

Winberg, J. (1999). Pacifier – partner or peril? *Acta Paediatrica*, **88**, 1177–9.

Winkelman, J. W., Herzog, D. B. & Fava, M. (1999). The prevalence of sleep-related eating disorder in psychiatric and nonpsychiatric populations. *Psychological Medicine*, **29**, 1461–6.

Wirz-Justice, A. & Van den Hoofdakker, R. H. (1999). Sleep deprivation in depression: what do we know, where do we go? *Biological Psychiatry*, **46**, 445–53.

Wolfson, A. R. & Carskadon, M. A. (1998). Sleep schedules and daytime functioning in adolescents. *Child Development*, **69**, 875–87.

Wolfson, A., Lacks, P. & Futterman, A. (1992). Effects of parent training on infant sleeping patterns, parents' stress and perceived parental control. *Journal of Consulting and Clinical Psychology*, **60**, 41–8.

Wszolek, Z. K., Groover, R. V. & Klass, D. W. (1995). Seizures presenting as episodic hypersomnolence. *Epilepsia*, **36**, 108–10.

Zai, C., Wigg, K. G. & Barr, C. L. (2000). Genetics and sleep disorders. *Seminars in Clinical Neuropsychiatry*, **5**, 33–43.

Zamir, G., Press, J., Tal, A. & Tarasiuk, A. (1998). Sleep fragmentation in children with juvenile rheumatoid arthritis. *Journal of Rheumatology*, **25**, 1191–7.

Zhdanova, I. V. (2000). The role of melatonin in sleep and sleep disorders. In *Sleep Disorders and Neurological Disease*, ed. A. Culebras, pp. 137–57. New York: Marcel Dekker.

Zhdanova, I. V., Wurtman, R. J. & Wagstaff, J. (1999). Effects of a low dose of melatonin on sleep in children with Angelman syndrome. *Journal of Pediatric Endocrinology and Metabolism*, **12**, 57–67.

Index